MW01258626

FASTING
CANCER

FASTING CANCER

How Fasting and Nutritechnology
Are Creating a Revolution in Cancer
Prevention and Treatment

VALTER LONGO, PhD

In collaboration with
Alessandro Laviano, MD
Romina Inés Cervigni, PhD
Cristina Villa, PhD

Avery
an imprint of Penguin Random House
New York

AVERY

an imprint of Penguin Random House LLC
penguinrandomhouse.com

Copyright © 2025 by Create Cures Foundation
First published as *Il cancro a digiuno* in Italy, by Antonio Vallardi Editore, Milano, in 2021.
First American edition published by Avery, an imprint of Penguin Random House LLC, in 2025.

Text on pages 20–23 and 24 was previously published in *The Longevity Diet* by the author.

Penguin Random House values and supports copyright. Copyright fuels creativity, encourages diverse voices, promotes free speech, and creates a vibrant culture. Thank you for buying an authorized edition of this book and for complying with copyright laws by not reproducing, scanning, or distributing any part of it in any form without permission. You are supporting writers and allowing Penguin Random House to continue to publish books for every reader. Please note that no part of this book may be used or reproduced in any manner for the purpose of training artificial intelligence technologies or systems.

Most Avery books are available at special quantity discounts for bulk purchase for sales promotions, premiums, fundraising, and educational needs. Special books or book excerpts also can be created to fit specific needs. For details, write SpecialMarkets@penguinrandomhouse.com.

Library of Congress Cataloging-in-Publication Data has been applied for.
ISBN (hardcover) 9780593545324
ISBN (e-book) 9780593545331

All illustrations are by Gilda Nappo, except for Illustration 5.1, made by Manuela Lupis and edited by Gilda Nappo.
Picture 2.2 taken from "Evolutionary Medicine: From Dwarf Model Systems to Healthy Centenarians?" by Valter Longo, Caleb E. Finch, published in *Science*, February 28, 2003: vol. 299, no. 5611.
Picture 2.4 © 2014 by Valter Longo.
Images on pages 86 and 150 from Ligorio et al., *European Journal of Cancer*, 2022.

Book design by Angie Boutin

Printed in the United States of America
1st Printing

Neither the publisher nor the author is engaged in rendering professional advice or services to the individual reader. The ideas, procedures, and suggestions contained in this book are not intended as a substitute for consulting with your physician. All matters regarding your health require medical supervision. Neither the author nor the publisher shall be liable or responsible for any loss or damage allegedly arising from any information or suggestion in this book.

While the author has made every effort to provide accurate telephone numbers, Internet addresses, and other contact information at the time of publication, neither the publisher nor the author assumes any responsibility for errors, or for changes that occur after publication. Further, the publisher does not have any control over and does not assume any responsibility for author or third-party websites or their content.

NOTE ABOUT THE DATA IN THIS BOOK

Data described in this book have been obtained from currently on-going animal or clinical studies. Therefore, beginning cycles of a fasting-mimicking diet is advised *only* after evaluation by and under the careful supervision of a patient's own specialized doctor and oncologist. It is extremely important to avoid malnutrition, a negative prognostic factor in both acute and chronic disease, but also to ensure that this and other nutritional interventions are appropriate considering the type and stage of cancer and the therapy to be administered (see appendix 1).

NOTE FROM THE AUTHOR

The Longevity and Healthspan Clinics of the Create Cures Foundation in the United States and the Valter Longo Foundation in Europe specialize in assisting patients and physicians in integrating standard approaches with innovative, evidence-based interventions. We focus on nutrition and molecular biology but also on the body's natural ability to fight cancer and other diseases. The foundations' mission is to help everyone live long and healthy. With available funding, assistance is offered at a discounted rate or free of charge to those who suffer from advanced-stage cancer and other pathologies and who cannot afford these integrated cures. I do not take a salary from L-Nutra, which I founded, and in addition I will continue to donate my shares of the company to research and charity. I also donate all of the earnings from my books to the Create Cures Foundation and the Valter Longo Foundation.

*To all the patients fighting for an opportunity
to beat cancer and live a long life*

CONTENTS

PREFACE

In 2012, *The New England Journal of Medicine*, considered by many to be the leading medical journal in the world, asked me to assess a scientific article regarding experimental models of neoplasm (an abnormal growth of cells that can be either benign or malignant).

The article in question demonstrated that rational and well-timed use of fasting was able to reduce the growth of cancer cells and increase receptivity to chemotherapy. In particular, the editors of the medical journal were interested in understanding whether the results obtained by testing mice and neoplastic cells could eventually be obtained in cancer patients. In short, I was being asked to predict the future with a crystal ball made up of complex mechanisms dictated by metabolism and immune system. I was already aware of this branch of research and the team that spearheaded it, namely that of Professor Valter Longo. However, this was my opportunity to study more in depth the reasons and workings of this innovative approach to treating neoplastic disease.

I must confess the medical horizon appeared hostile to the inclusion of fasting or fasting-mimicking diets in treatment for cancer patients. In general, we, doctors and oncologists included, receive a drug-focused training and therefore focus on administering drugs to treat illnesses. We know little about the powerful metabolic effects of food and fasting, so we find it hard to admit they play a role in treating patients diagnosed with cancer. In addition, my medical and scientific training was directed at preventing and treating malnutrition in cancer patients. For this reason, at first glance, my clinical and scientific capabilities seemed to be not only estranged from the fasting method used in oncology but downright antithetical. I still remember the reaction to Professor Longo's address when he spoke at the 2012 European Society for Clinical Nutrition and Metabolism Congress in Barcelona. While I was not present for his speech, I heard about the furious discussions during the Q&A session, with most in the room strongly believing patients should be fed a lot of food during treatment. Maybe the heated exchange was the reason that Professor Longo did not attend the social dinner later that evening, in the fear of his plate being laced with some form of cathartic drug. (In truth, Valter has always told me he did not attend simply because he lost the invitation card.)

Science, especially medical science, proceeds by hypothesis, verifications, and possible successes. This means that everlasting dogmas, in every corner of the universe, cannot exist. Universal laws can be drawn only in physics. Therefore, the best way to allow medical research to evolve, with its patients' well-being in mind, is to not accept the concept of ipse dixit, of an inflexible and immovable authority, but constantly ask oneself questions with a curious and critical spirit in the face of evidence, however counterintuitive it may be. With this spirit in mind, when I was rereading the article in *The New England Journal of Medicine*, two key points were clear to me: (1) the scientific evidence presented was more than solid; (2) in cancer patients, it is possible to hypothesize a synergy between protection of the nutritional status and the fasting-mimicking diet, where the former is aimed at safely implementing the latter. I concluded my readings with "cautious optimism" and trust in the clinical studies being conducted at the time to test the efficiency of fasting and a fasting-mimicking diet.

Thirteen years have gone by since then, and the role of fasting and the fasting-mimicking diet is no longer a taboo in treatment of patients. Experimental studies conducted years ago are now supported by clinical data in both healthy people and cancer patients. Some cancer centers are already open to the integration of traditional therapy and metabolic therapy, at least for some types of cancer. Furthermore, the overall scenario for the fight against cancer has become more complex and requires innovative strategies. It is evident that many antineoplastic drugs, i.e., anticancer drugs, have a reduced efficiency compared with what was shown in studies performed to request approval from regulatory authorities (for example, the Food and Drug Administration [FDA] in the United States and the European Medicines Agency [EMA] in Europe); such approval of a drug is necessary before it can be put on the market. Many new drugs are extremely expensive but also require improvements of their effectiveness profile. Lastly, recent statistics seem to underline a progressive reduction in the cancer mortality rate but simultaneously an increase in long-term side effects due to cancer and perhaps to therapy itself. This scenario brings to the forefront the importance of the patient's quality of life, a parameter that is often forgotten or undermined in the approval of new drugs.

This book is not intended to represent new guidelines in cancer treatment. Rather, its objective is to simply pay tribute to the work of a group of scientists in recent years that has led to great promise for cancer patients. The scientific evidence on fasting and fasting-mimicking diet is solid and concrete but undoubtedly does not yet allow them to be included in standard-of-care therapies. It does, however, allow them to be considered for integration into standard therapy, especially when there are no alternatives proven to be effective. In consideration of the metabolic power of fasting and food, the recommendation is to decide whether to follow this option only after having discussed it with an oncologist. Fasting and the fasting-mimicking diet in oncology are not panaceas and remedies for all ailments, and they do not guarantee control or regression of the disease. The book discusses how clinical responses vary depending on the cancer type and patient. Therefore, integrating clinically tested fasting-mimicking diets under medical supervision into standard-of-care therapies should be considered an option that allows for an increase in one's own chances of reaping benefits from antineoplastic drugs. And whereas we may not think a 5 percent discount is a big deal at the grocery store, for a cancer patient a chance of recovery that is increased by 5 percent could be lifesaving, literally.

I would like to end on a more personal note. After the article's publication, I met Professor Longo in person, and we began collaborating and became good friends. I believe in Valter, and I share the thought that a profitable collaboration is based on the recognition and respect of each other's capabilities. As in life, diversity and respect help to achieve great results. I am convinced of the potential of integrating fasting and the fasting-mimicking diet in the treatment of cancer patients and those affected by other diseases, but only clinical trials can provide conclusive results on the matter, which is why our efforts continue.

Alessandro Laviano
Associate Professor of Medicine in the Department of
Translational and Precision Medicine
at Sapienza University of Rome, Italy

FASTING
CANCER

INTRODUCTION

In 2019, a young female patient came to the foundation clinic and told me she had advanced-stage breast cancer, possibly incurable. Her initial meeting with an oncologist had been brief and hurried, and she was hoping that I could help further. As a biochemist, a cancer researcher, and a juventologist (someone who studies the health span in efforts to maintain youth), I started to think about whether the cancer in that woman was unavoidable. Why did she— and nearly half of the U.S. and European population—get cancer at all? I was well aware that mice, whose life span is about two and a half years, would start to develop tumors around one and a half years of age, but *people* rarely developed tumors at that age. So cancer depended not on time but on the aging and life span phase of the organism. Aging was by far the major risk factor for most cancers in both mice and humans, so I knew that we should focus on aging to prevent cancer. But why was everyone talking about preventing cancer, if aging was by far the major risk factor for cancer?

I often start a medical presentation by asking the audience, "How much longer do you think we would live on average if we completely cured cancer today?" The answers range from ten to twenty-five years. Everyone is very surprised when I tell them, "Sadly, it's only three to four years longer." Recently, I pointed this out to one of the most famous cancer scientists on the planet, who responded, "Then shall we all stop cancer research and go home?" As someone who spends half of his time focusing on cancer research at the USC Norris Cancer Center in L.A. and the IFOM Institute of Molecular Oncology in Milan, Italy, I was trying to make the point that we should concentrate less specifically on cancer prevention and start focusing more on slowing the aging process, since it is a major risk factor for many diseases and dysfunctions, not just cancer.

At another conference, someone raised their hand and relayed to the audience, "I knew a lady who every morning around eleven used to drink a glass of grappa [a grape-based distilled spirit from Italy]. Then one day she moved into a nursing home, and when she turned one hundred and three, they told her that for health reasons she could no longer have the grappa. Shortly after, she died." Everyone laughed and expected me to defend the decision of taking away the grappa, but they were surprised when I said light alcohol consumption (up to a few drinks per week) has either a neutral or a slightly positive association with longevity. A journalist moderating the interview pointed out that alcohol should be completely avoided by everyone, since it is a cancer risk factor. But that isn't accurate: although alcohol is a risk factor for certain cancers, the effect of low alcohol consumption on the risk for most cancers is either very small or null. We should be focusing on how alcohol affects juventology and health span, not just cancer. Yes, a certain food or drink could cause a slight increase in the risk of developing cancer, but it could also have protective effects against diabetes, cardiovascular disease, or Alzheimer's, or it could simply make the person much happier and willing to fight to live longer and healthier. That food or drink can still be recommended to most people but should be avoided by someone at high risk for developing one of the tumors affected by alcohol (for example, head and neck cancers).[1]

We need to treat aging or, better yet, promote youth span (the period of life during which a person remains young) and health span. But this is not as easy as it seems. Just like the decision whether to drink alcohol, the decision to follow a specific diet must be based on multiple factors. Take, for instance, Emma Morano from Verbania, Italy, whom I followed for the last five years of her life. She called her doctor, Carlo Bava, when she was over 100 (she lived until 117, the oldest person in the world when she died) and told him she thought she should stop eating red meat. Dr. Bava asked why, and she replied, "A journalist told me that it causes cancer." While meat consumption is a risk factor for cancer, it should have been a secondary worry for the centenarian Morano. For years to come, cancer will be one of the most common and lethal diseases worldwide, and adopting a diet that delays aging and prevents obesity will be the best way to avoid it. The Longevity Diet was created with this in mind; and its recommendations should be tailored to each person and their specific age. For example, the centenarian Emma might have benefited by eating red meat to avoid malnutrition, which is a major risk factor for older adults, and not worrying so much about its associations with cancer. Someone who is forty-five, on the other hand, should be more concerned with both the prevention of cancer and malnutrition factors. Additionally, finding the right team to implement antiaging and cancer strategies can be the difference between life and death for many people, as it was for Emma, who found Dr. Bava.

According to the American Cancer Society, people in the U.S. have about a 40 percent risk of developing cancer and a 20 percent risk of dying from it.[2] This is not just an American problem, since the numbers are similar in Europe. Cancer Research UK reports that about 50 percent of people living there will be diagnosed with cancer in their lifetime.[3] In Italy, the Italian Association of Medical Oncology (AIOM) in collaboration with the Italian Association of Cancer Registries (ARTIUM) determined that 50 percent of men (one in two) and more than 30 percent of women (one in three) are likely to be diagnosed with cancer.[4]

One wonders how we have been so successful in reducing the risk of cardiovascular and many other diseases but have had very limited success with cancer. The answer lies in the molecular mechanisms responsible:

1. Cancer can start in most cell types and organs, giving rise to forms of the disease that share some similarities but also have major differences.
2. A tumor mass does not include a single cancer cell type but rather many types, each of which could respond, or not, to a particular therapy.
3. Even if a cancer therapy is effective against 99.9 percent of cancer cells, those one in one thousand cancer cells that do survive can generate new masses, which are often more difficult to fight than the original ones.
4. Tumor masses can contain cancer stem cells, which can continue to generate new cancer cells even if the therapy appears to be effective.
5. It is relatively easy to kill cancer cells, but it is much more difficult to kill cancer cells without killing or damaging normal cells.

The standard cancer therapies, ranging from chemotherapy and immunotherapy to hormone therapy, need improvement, particularly in being effective against a wider range of cancer cells, in killing cancer stem cells, in preventing cells from becoming resistant to the therapy, and in preserving normal cells. Fasting and nutrition may have the highest potential to provide this type of integrative approach to cancer treatment, at least for the foreseeable future.

AN "UNCONSPIRED CONSPIRACY"

Why are so many people getting cancer? The answer lies in part in what I call an "unconspired conspiracy." We have known for years that a Western diet rich in calories from animal fat, proteins, refined carbs, and sugars can lead to obesity and cardiovascular disease in addition to increasing the risk for cancer and neurodegeneration. Yet food companies, pharmaceutical companies, the media, hospitals, clinics, and doctors participate in this unconspired conspiracy by going along and promoting the status quo. It is "unconspired" because there is no outright collusion between the food industry that sells unhealthy processed foods, candy, or sugary drinks and the pharmaceutical companies selling drugs to treat nutrition-related diseases like diabetes and heart conditions. In addition, the great majority of doctors have good intentions, and they don't have many alternatives for treatment other than prescribing those medications. As I discussed in my first book, *The Longevity Diet*, the solution is clear: to improve your health, adopt a diet and lifestyle that increase your chances of a long, healthy life. This is based not on my opinion but on hundreds of studies related to the five solid pillars of longevity (epidemiology, clinical trials, basic research focused on longevity, studies of centenarians, and studies of complex systems).

The science is clear, yet the world is slow to change and collect the benefits in terms of health, life span, and financial savings (the U.S. spends nearly 20 percent of its GDP on health care). Why?

1. Most doctors are trained for sick care. They usually receive only one course on nutrition in medical school, so they are not taught how diet can promote a healthy longevity or how to get patients to adopt and maintain a longevity lifestyle.

2. Some food and drug companies benefit from "information confusion"—the persistent and contradicting data on what foods are healthy and unhealthy—and are able to push drugs as the primary way to treat a condition or disease. They pay thousands of academic consultants and fund the many commercials and ads you encounter daily. Not all companies do this; there are many that promote healthy foods and create remarkable drugs. And I

am not against drug therapy; I am only against those that are ineffective or merely put a Band-Aid on a problem that may be better served by nutritional and other lifestyle changes.

3. Hospitals and clinics can make much more money if people are chronically sick than if they live a disease-free life. It may not be intentional, but there is no incentive to cure people.

4. Scientists frequently use a one-pillar strategy (for example, a focus on epidemiology) and are often steeped in their own world of research and academia. While it is critical that scientists be focused on their basic research, this often comes at a price to the patients. While this strategy is great for the advancement of science, it's terrible for people who are sick, at least in the short term. The solution is for scientists to be part of the treatment team together with doctors and nutrition experts.

5. The media is often confused by all of the above and is worried about backlash from food companies, drug companies, and the medical community alike.

It's an unconspired conspiracy because everyone, including me, is going along with a system that keeps us employed and makes many companies and hospitals rich. So who is responsible? We all are. We are in dire need of academic sources of information we can trust; doctors who are properly trained in nutrition and health span; hospitals that truly care about helping people become healthy and stay that way; and food and nutritechnology companies (like the ones I founded) that focus on the health and longevity of their customers and on the environment without making money a major factor. (To reduce the conflict of interest that affects so many professionals in the health-care field, I do not take a consulting fee or a salary from L-nutra, and I have pledged to donate 95 percent of my shares to research and charity, with the remaining 5 percent to be invested in socially and environmentally responsible companies.)

TEAMS OF DOCTORS AND BIOLOGISTS

This same mission-based mentality should be applied to everyone, and nutrition and fasting held as central pillars. Unfortunately, in recent years we have grown progressively more concerned with our positions on health: lifestyle versus genetics, vegan or carnivore, traditional or alternative medicine. If we could move away from this us-versus-them mentality and concentrate on the fundamentals of health and longevity, while keeping in mind tradition, history, and the effect of dietary choices on pollution and the environment, we could achieve much more at a lower cost. For example, someone who likes meat may belong to the carnivore ideology and refuse to acknowledge any of its negative effects, whereas a vegan may refuse to acknowledge that some vegans may experience malnourishment. If we instead focus on the mission, we can help people find a path to live longer and healthier regardless of ideology.

Consequently, a mission-based and problem-solving approach is essential. I want to stress the importance of building clinics with multidisciplinary medical teams including physicians, molecular biologists,[5] dietitians, psychologists, and other specialties working together to solve complex medical problems. In our Los Angeles Create Cures Foundation Clinic, registered dietitians are working closely with physicians and molecular biologists, as well as with external specialists treating cancer, diabetes, cardiovascular disease, neurodegeneration, autoimmunities, and other diseases, many at advanced stages. I have to admit that the initial phases were challenging for everyone. We wrestled with determining the role of each member of the team. I had to reassure the medical doctors that they were in charge of any decision related to disease treatment and how much time they should spend with their patients, but we slowly overcame these challenges and are now beginning to publish studies on the efficacy of the teams, the Longevity Diet, fasting-mimicking diets, and other science-based nutritional or integrative interventions on patients with a range of diseases.

OLD CANCER THERAPY
VERSUS NEW CANCER THERAPY

Years ago, when I was attending one of the largest cancer confer-
ences in the world, I noticed the organizers didn't have any sessions dedicated to side effects of cancer therapy. So I proposed to
organize one in the next conference; they turned down my request,
even though the influential conference did not have a single part
dedicated to patient protection. This sort of thinking represents the
old cancer-therapy model based mostly on the magic bullet (chemotherapy, immunotherapy, etc.) to kill cancer cells. We should
reconsider this outdated mentality and instead provide patients
with the type of 360-degree care and multidisciplinary team that
can maximize the chance of a cure but also improve healthy longevity. In this book I talk about not only how nutrition and fasting-
mimicking diets can lead to better care but also the right type of
medical team and system to optimize the therapy. For what I call
the "Longevity Revolution" to be successful, the doctors must wel-
come it, dietitians working with these doctors need to implement
it, and companies need to develop new products or services that
will help people have longer and healthier lives while simultaneously generating revenue.

Why is a 360-degree care method implemented by a multidisciplinary team necessary, particularly in the cancer-treatment
setting? Because each cancer has a molecular weakness and all
cancers require lots of nutrients to grow, but they also continue to
change. For this reason, fighting cancer with only one or a few
drugs is like fighting a war by employing only the infantry. We
need to fight tactically by thinking differently about the problem.
While cancer can be attacked frontally with chemotherapy or radiation, we also need the immune system to attack the cancer cells,
all the while ensuring minimal damage to the normal cells and
organs of the body. To do this, we need to exploit the fact that normal cells and cancer cells can have very different needs for a particular amino acid, sugar, fat, or growth factor. The cancer cells

may need high levels of sugar, whereas the normal cells are fine with relatively low blood-sugar levels. This is where nutrition and evolutionary biology meet oncology. In our research, we found a way to exploit those needs through a combination of standard therapy and a fasting-mimicking diet—one that "tricks" your body into responding as if it is fasting but allows some food intake, providing the right amount of nutrients and calories. Studies have shown that fasting-mimicking diets seem to protect normal cells while cancer cells become more vulnerable to many therapies ranging from chemo to radiation, immunotherapy, and hormone therapy. While we have learned that you cannot starve cancer with fasting alone, since cancer steals from other cells and finds a way to stay alive even if the patient fasts, you can use fasting-mimicking diets to make the cancer cells so weak or desperate that the right therapy will kill them. These nutrition-based interventions are exploiting the differences in the biochemistry and molecular biology of normal and cancer cells.

All this is to say, that the types of standard and integrative therapies used can make the difference between whether someone dies at twenty-five of a lymphoma (a blood cancer), dies at thirty-two of an adenocarcinoma (for example, breast cancer), or lives disease free to one hundred. Integrative therapies (therapies added to the standard cancer treatment) do have the potential to make a big difference for cancer patients. This approach can also help us all have a better chance of overcoming most diseases and achieving a healthier life span. But we are waging a tough battle. Most oncologists consider any nutrition-based therapy "quackery," in many cases without even having read and understood the basis for this therapy. In their defense, they are so busy practicing that they often don't have the time to investigate every idea brought to them by patients or scientists. However, with advanced-stage cancers for which there is no effective therapy, the oncologist should take the time to learn about integrative therapies that have sufficient laboratory and clinical evidence to be considered safe and potentially effective. For instance, most mainstream doctors write off vitamin C therapy, but high doses of the vitamin injected in combination with the fasting-mimicking diet have been shown to be effective in animal studies.[6] In an ideal situation, an open-minded oncologist treating a KRAS-mutated colon cancer patient who has run out of effective therapies could discuss the vitamin C studies with their patient and, based on local law, could combine injectable vitamin C with the fasting-mimicking diet and standard treatment. They could also take advantage of the "compassionate use" rule.

Compassionate use, according to the FDA, "is a potential pathway for a patient with an immediately life-threatening condition or serious disease to gain access to an investigational medical product (drug, biologic, or medical device) for treatment outside of clinical trials when no comparable or satisfactory alternative therapy options are available."[7] This is a high hurdle for the doctor to clear, but it can potentially make a big difference for the patient, as we will see in the following chapters. In Italy, at various leading cancer centers in collaboration with my group and the Creates Cures Foundation clinics, we have introduced these types of integrative interventions as part of an open feasibility clinical trial that has enrolled many patients with a wide range of tumors. This approach, based on clinical protocols that have been approved by ethical committees, is ideal until the integrative therapy becomes standard. However, starting clinical trials is very difficult for the great majority of oncologists and therefore is rarely done, making "compassionate use" an important alternative.

THIS BOOK

This book focuses on the tremendous potential and effectiveness of fasting-mimicking diets and the Longevity Diet in combination with standard cancer therapy, as well as their prevention and mitigation of side effects. The research is ongoing, but this book is based on thirty years of aging studies and twenty years of cancer studies carried out by my laboratories and many others in the U.S. and Europe, as well as on the many clinical trials at some of the best hospitals, to address both cancer prevention and cancer treatment while focusing on the "patient first."

The early chapters on cancer prevention are straightforward, since they are mostly focused on nutrition and healthy longevity. Nevertheless, the recommendations included are not as obvious as one might think, because they must achieve antiaging/anticancer effects while avoiding malnourishment and frailty, including the loss of bone, muscle, and immune function. It's important that people continue to enjoy the food they eat and implement limited changes that they can easily keep up for the rest of their lives. It is not about improvised advice we hear every day, such as "Eat less or eat in moderation" or "Eat like your grandma" or "Eat like people in the Paleolithic period" or "Eat low carb" or even "Eat the Mediterranean diet." It is about eating a personalized diet with a sufficient but limited number of ingredients that you like and enjoy and that allow you to maintain a normal weight and fat mass. It is also about understanding that obesity and insulin resistance are modern conditions arising from normal states evolved to survive long winters or periods of starvation. This knowledge and its evolutionary and molecular foundation can be used to optimize healthy longevity and help prevent cancer.

I focus the lion's share of the book on different cancers, their origins, and the studies conducted on various treatments in tandem with the fasting-mimicking diet and other nutrition-based interventions. While this is challenging, as we continue to do research, I'm confident that one day we can cure many cancers via therapies that include fasting-mimicking diets and other interventions that make cancer cells much more sensitive to therapy and normal cells much more resistant to therapies. Since we already know how to do this in microorganisms and mice, this goal is achievable.

We know that nutritional interventions that accompany standard-of-care treatments have central roles in how effective the treatment is. In fact, we have known some of this for a hundred years, since Otto Warburg described how cancer cells are avid consumers of sugars and producers of lactic acid, a finding that contributed to his 1923 Nobel Prize now called "the Warburg effect" (see chapter 7). But reducing glucose or even fasting is not enough, as we will see in most of the cancer chapters. This book is not about overriding or dismissing the remarkable and often heroic work done by oncologists; rather it is about giving oncologists additional tools and motivation to help incurable patients. I also hope it can help them decrease short-term and long-term side effects, especially when viable alternatives are not available.

FOR THOSE INTERESTED IN PREVENTING cancer (and a number of other diseases), this book will offer guidance on slowing down aging and reducing biological age. It won't always be easy, but the great majority of people can understand and follow these guidelines. If you have been diagnosed with cancer or have had cancer in the past, our teams at the nonprofit Create Cures Foundation Clinic in the U.S. and at the Valter Longo Foundation Clinics in Europe are ready to help you implement what I discuss in the book. I also encourage you to find oncologists who are open-minded and willing to go out of their way to make sure you not only beat cancer but also prevent long-lasting side effects and increase your probability of making it to one hundred healthy.

1

FASTING CANCER, FEEDING PATIENTS

TO DEFEAT YOUR ENEMY, KNOW HIM WELL

It was 1994 and I was a second-year pathology PhD student in the UCLA laboratory headed by Roy Walford, MD, one of the leading experts in calorie-restriction studies, when I found out I was not made for "close contact" medicine. One day, while I was taking a pathology course, the chief pathologist started handing me the body parts of a forty-five-year-old male who had just died of cancer, asking me, "What do you see?" I was not pursuing a medical degree like his medical students, so he was pushing me, hoping that I would get sick and run out. Nevertheless, I had just completed five years of brutal treatment as a tanker in the U.S. Army Reserve and I was not about to give him the satisfaction, so I looked at the dead body, then looked at the lungs in my hands and, without flinching, went on to tell him whatever insignificant observations a second-year graduate student could give him.

That patient, a forty-five-year-old smoker, had died of lung cancer, and that situation affected me a lot more than I wanted to admit. It affected me because of how young he was, because of the smell in that room, and because in the moment the chief pathologist placed his lungs in my hands, I knew how fragile life was, what our research was all about, and how important it was to focus, to think differently, to have a mission, and not to go to work just because I wanted to be a successful scientist. That man would probably have still been alive had someone been able to tell him how to prevent that cancer by quitting smoking or maybe adopting a nutritional program to better protect him from the harm of cigarettes. He might also have been alive if immunotherapy or a fasting-mimicking-diet-based therapy had been implemented thirty years ago. In addition to the psychological effect, I did not eat for two days, did not eat meat for weeks, and was on my way to becoming a pescatarian.

The cancer that had killed my grandfather by generating a metastatic intestinal tumor had also killed this forty-five-year-old man, and it was now my enemy. I was in one of the best cancer centers and hospitals in the world, and most young researchers would have stayed right there, in the perfect place to work on aging and cancer. However, my instinct told me that this enemy had much deeper molecular secrets than those investigated in the pathology department. I had to understand where it came from, how it evolved, and why it behaved in a certain way. I thought about my summer work on starving bacteria in the laboratory of Steven Clarke in the biochemistry department before I moved to pathology in 1992, and I decided to go back to that department and work with two exceptional women (Joan Valentine and Edie Gralla) to get to know an organism that's a little closer to human beings than bacteria are: the baker's yeast *Saccharomyces cerevisiae*. It is more similar to humans because, although it is a single-cell organism, it is a eukaryote just like us; in other words, it is an organism whose cells have a nucleus within a nuclear membrane.

I went back to the biochemistry department, and within months I observed something very strange: the yeasts died, but then they appeared to come back to life (figure 1.1).

· · · · · · ·

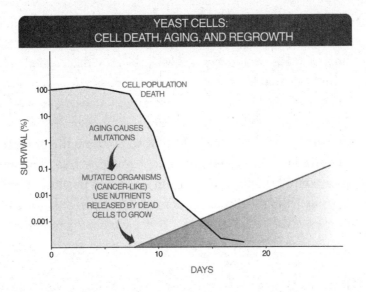

1.1. *As the yeast grows, it ages, which causes mutations in its DNA. Similar to what happens in cancer cells, some of these mutations can give the altered organisms the capacity to use the nutrients left behind by the dead ones in order to grow. The population then "regenerates" itself, because although some organisms die, others proliferate. Modified from Paola Fabrizio et al., "Superoxide Is a Mediator of an Altruistic Aging Program in Saccharomyces Cerevisiae,"* Journal of Cell Biology *166, no. 7 (2004): 1055–67.*

WHAT IS CANCER?

Later I will discuss the yeast experiment above and the potential origin of cancer, but it is important first to explain what cancer is. Contrary to the widely disseminated opinion that cancer cells are smart and powerful, most are actually confused and weak, but they can grow fast or grow when they are not supposed to. Within the large group of cancer cells in a tumor mass, some can survive and continue to grow, thus making cancer very difficult to fight. What are the features of cancer cells that make them "confused" but also deadly? Douglas Hanahan and Robert Weinberg described them in a famous article entitled "Hallmarks of Cancer," originally published in 2000 and expanded since.[1]

- **Sustained proliferation.** The great majority of cancer cells can continue to proliferate in places where and when normal cells would not grow. This growth is aided by mutations that keep certain growth genes always on: the oncogenes (genes that have the potential to cause cancer). The normal, nonmutated versions of oncogenes, proto-oncogenes (such as RAS, AKT, PKA), promote the growth of cells but also accelerate aging. Imagine that the gas pedal in your car is damaged and won't ease up; now imagine this happening in a city, on narrow streets chock-full of cars. And imagine that for every car that gets into an accident and stops, one or two more enter the roadway. Clearly, devastation is ahead.

- **Evasion of growth suppressors.** Tumor-suppressor genes are designed to prevent the oncogenes, which are the modified genes that promote cancer growth, and other factors from generating cancer cells. Their job includes preventing the cell from dividing (to generate another cell) but also killing cells that have been damaged enough to present a danger to the rest of the organism. Think of tumor-suppressor genes as the rough equivalent of car brake pedals; mutations of these genes cause the brakes to no longer work.

- **Invasion and metastasis.** Normally, normal cells remain within a certain tissue because they receive mechanical signals (they are pushed or blocked by other cells) and are exposed to factors that suppress their growth and relocation. Cancer cells instead disobey these orders and invade tissues and areas that are normally off-limits to them. One invasion that makes them particularly dangerous is that of blood vessels, which, using the car analogy, are like highways that allow the cancer cells to reach distant sites in a process called metastasis. Once the cancer advances to this level, it becomes much more difficult to treat, as each metastasized cancer cell can also acquire new mutations and/or features.

- **Circumvention of replicative senescence.** In addition to tumor-suppressor genes, normal cells also have a cell-division clock that sets a limit on the number of times a cell can reproduce. Known as replicative senescence, this clock is controlled in part by the length of telomeres, the pieces of DNA found on each end of a chromosome. If these telomeres are long enough, the cell can continue to generate new cells. But telomeres shorten as we age, halting cell growth. At this point the cell is considered senescent or, simply, old. Cancer cells can get around this hurdle by activating an enzyme called telomerase, which keeps telomeres from shrinking and allows the cancer cell to continue growing.
- **Refusing death.** Once they are damaged, normal cells are programmed to die via a process called apoptosis. Many cancer cells, however, have the ability to block this mechanism. Certain cancer drugs target this override feature, thereby killing the cells.

In addition to these traditional features of cancer cells, we have learned that they can also thrive in the presence of inflammation, and that they acquire defenses against immune cells to avoid being targeted for destruction. Finally, because of their ability to quickly mutate and evolve, some cancer cells within a cancer mass can escape aggressive treatment and survive.

THE ORIGIN OF CANCER?

When I showed the apparent baker's yeast–resuscitation experiment (figure 1.1) to my mentors, they were puzzled. How did the yeast come back to life or grow so rapidly if we did not give them any food? The answer required ten years of research and was published in 2004, after I became a professor at USC School of Gerontology, a center famous for its research on aging. As the yeast organisms were aging and dying according to an "altruistic death program" (whereby organisms die for the sake of other organisms), they generated many DNA mutations, a few of which enabled them to thrive and grow in the food-limited environment. Those with the "growth mutations" were able to feed off the nutrients released by the dead and dying yeast to keep growing. Was this struggle to adapt and survive the origin of cancer?

Just like cancer cells, the yeast cells were not thwarted by the starvation conditions that would normally signal cells to stop growing. This could represent a very early example of mutations causing a "cancer-like" growth in yeast cells, which are called oncogenes in mammals, with central roles in human cancer. So this phenomenon suggests that cancer may represent an evolution of mutations in certain growth genes (the oncogenes) that originally allowed unicellular organisms to adapt and grow in otherwise hostile environments. This process is normally inactive in human cells but may be activated by mistake due to aging or other factors like carcinogens.

Thus, human mutations leading to cancer are random and arise from age-dependent mishandling of processes that have a biological role. For example, free radicals that are produced during the normal function of a cell can cause damage to DNA and trigger mutations that could favor the formation of cancer cells. One important aspect of oncogene mutations, which I will discuss again later in the book, is that they often occur in a limited number of genetic pathways (IGF-1R, RAS, PKA, AKT) that also accelerate the aging process and, when inactivated, make different types of organisms live longer.

MORE AND MORE CONFUSED CELLS

Cancer cells are equipped with mutations and other changes that make them excellent at growing but also able to survive under unfavorable conditions. Furthermore, because they are always stuck in an accelerated-aging mode, they generate massive damage to DNA and cellular components, making them in many cases progressively more suited to grow and survive only as long as all the necessary nutrients are available. In fact, whereas all or at least the great majority of normal cells in a human body can adjust to the limitations of all external nutrients, the cancer cells do not have this ability or it is strongly impaired. They become progressively more dependent on receiving excess quantities of nutrients from the patient.

But what does virtually every hospital do? They make cancer patients eat *more* food, in the hope that this will compensate for the muscle and weight loss caused by the cancer and requisite therapy. Although this overfeeding can, in many cases, benefit the muscle mass or weight of the patient, the research indicates it will benefit cancer cells the most. If we consider that it takes about two months of starvation from a complete lack of food for humans to begin to die, it is clear that most, if not all, cancer cells would also die after prolonged periods of fasting in combination with therapy. The very challenging goal is to kill all the cancer cells before hurting the patient and, just as important, before weakening the systems crucial to fighting the cancer, such as the immune system and the nervous system.

THE MAGIC SHIELD

Years after completing my PhD at UCLA, I met a child with an advanced-stage neuroblastoma at Children's Hospital Los Angeles. Neuroblastoma is a type of cancer that forms from immature nerve cells and starts in the adrenal glands on the top of the kidneys or abdomen, in the chest, and in nerve tissue near the spine. This encounter in the early 2000s, when we were doing research on aging, not cancer, made me think about my days in the pathology department at UCLA and the autopsy of that forty-five-year-old man who died of cancer. I realized that we were experts in "stress resistance," the genes and processes that make a cell more protected against toxins, such as free radicals and other cancer-causing substances. I also realized that the oncology researchers had a deep understanding of how DNA mutations and cellular damage affect cancer cells but almost no knowledge of or interest in how to protect normal cells. Because we had just discovered that the oncogenes that give cancer cells the ability to disobey orders and continue growing also make them weaker and more vulnerable to the damage caused by toxins, I speculated that maybe this was the first way to distinguish all normal cells from all cancer cells, and so I asked several researchers in my group to switch their focus to cancer research.

Paola Fabrizio, a postdoctoral fellow researcher in my group, and I coauthored a series of papers on studies using yeast as a model organism to identify which genes accelerate the aging process. Mario Mirisola, another researcher in my laboratory, helped me identify the link between genes that accelerate aging—making cells more vulnerable—and specific nutrients. Remarkably, these were the same genes central to cancer—oncogenes.

Every cancer researcher was looking for a "magic bullet" that would seek out and destroy only cancer cells. I remember in the early 2000s calling one of my colleagues, a famous scientist in the aging field, to float my theory. I told her, "I think I have figured out a way to distinguish all cancer cells from all normal cells. It is not a magic bullet—it is a magic shield." I don't think she had any idea what I was talking about and was not impressed.

What I proposed, and eventually called differential stress resistance, was based on the idea that, if you starve an organism, it will go into a highly protected, non-growth mode. This is the "shield," which is accompanied by the activation of protective enzymes like those that block oxidative damage (the damage that oxygen and similar molecules cause when they react with molecules, including those in DNA, proteins, or fats). However, a cancer cell will disobey this order and continue growing, even when it is starved, because the oncogene is stuck in an always-on mode (figure 1.2).

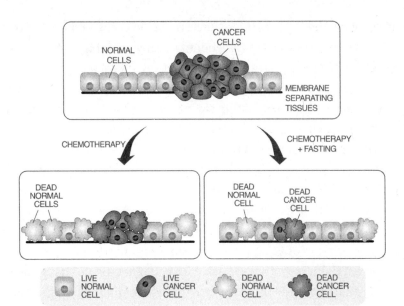

1.2. *Differential stress resistance is based on the different response, during starvation, of the normal cells compared with the cancer cells when under toxic therapies, including chemotherapy or radiation. During fasting, the normal cells either slow down or stop growing in order to protect themselves, creating a protective shield that allows them to survive with reduced levels of nutrients; cancer cells do not stop nor become protected. This renders cancer cells more sensitive to toxins. Modified from Alessio Nencioni et al., "Fasting and Cancer: Molecular Mechanisms and Clinical Application,"* Nature Reviews Cancer *18, no. 11 (2018): 707–19.*

Think about the Punic Wars and imagine a battlefield where ancient Romans and Carthaginians are mixed together wearing the same uniform. The common approach of cancer therapies is to seek a "magic arrow" (the bullet) that will kill only the Carthaginian soldiers, without harming the Romans. This is tricky, because the soldiers all look the same to archers standing one hundred yards away. However, before shooting their arrows, suppose the archers ordered the soldiers, in Latin, to kneel and raise their shields. Because only the Romans would understand the command, they would take cover, while the Carthaginians would remain standing and exposed to the incoming arrows. In this imaginary historical analogy, the Romans are the normal cells of the body, the Carthaginians the cancer cells, the archers the oncologists, and the arrows the chemotherapy. Notably, the Romans effectively used this strategy to protect themselves from the enemy's arrows and called it the "tortoise formation." If you starve a cancer patient before injecting chemotherapy, normal cells will respond by putting up a defensive shield. Nevertheless, cancer cells will ignore the command to protect themselves and thus remain vulnerable, providing a way to potentially eradicate cancer cells with minimal damage to normal cells.

To prove this, in a 2008 study, we took a yeast cell and generated an oncogene-like mutation called RASval19 in it, essentially producing a population of yeast cells that behaved like cancer cells. Then we mixed them in the same flask with cells that did not have oncogenes, and we treated them with various chemotherapy drugs. Even though the normal and the cancer-like yeast cells were mixed in the same flasks, just as normal and cancer cells are mixed together in the blood or tissues of patients, chemotherapy killed 100 percent of the cancer cells and spared all the normal cells (figure 1.3).

Our first cancer-related mouse study, for the same 2008 publication, was very simple—basically a spin-off of our experiment in microorganisms. For this, I asked Changhan Lee, one of my graduate students in the Los Angeles laboratory, and Lizzia Raffaghello, a researcher in Genoa, to perform a new, very unconventional experiment: switch mice with cancer to water-only fasting for two or three days before giving them multiple cycles of chemotherapy.

The results were stunning. Virtually all the fasting mice were alive and behaving normally after high-dose chemotherapy, while the mice on a normal diet were sick and lethargic after chemotherapy. In the following weeks, 65 percent of the mice that had not fasted died, whereas nearly all the fasted mice survived. We reproduced this same effect using a wide variety of chemotherapy drugs. As hoped and predicted, starvation consistently caused "multistress resistance," or protection against many different toxins, in normal cells but not in cancer cells, which were killed by the chemotherapy. We knew this approach had great clinical potential,

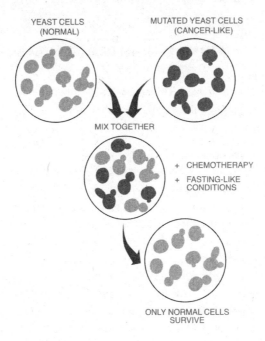

1.3. *The cancer-like yeast cells (mutated RASval19) behave differently from the normal cells when the two are mixed together and exposed to chemotherapy in conditions that mimic fasting. Chemotherapy kills 100 percent of cancer-like cells, sparing all normal cells. Modified from Lizzia Raffaghello et al., "Starvation-Dependent Differential Stress Resistance Protects Normal but Not Cancer Cells Against High-Dose Chemotherapy,"* Proceedings of the National Academy of Sciences of the United States of America *105, no. 24 (2008): 8215–20.*

but it still would not be easy to get the medical community to consider it.

CANCER REMISSION IN MICE

In 1812, Napoleon invaded Russia with more than 450,000 men. As the French, German, Austrian, Polish, and Italian army moved toward Moscow, the Russian forces didn't fight back. They retreated, burning their own villages and towns before the enemy's advance. Napoleon was surprised and confused. The invasion had started in June, but the Russians refused to fight until December. The strategic retreat was meant to weaken Napoleon's army.

TO ANIMAL-RIGHTS ACTIVISTS

I occasionally receive emails from animal-rights activists wondering why mice must suffer and die for the sake of research. Here is my answer:

- We work as much as possible with cells and microorganisms. Nevertheless, it is important, even essential, to test interventions in mice before any human clinical trial, in order to improve our research and help patients all over the world. In most cases human clinical trials are not allowed in the absence of animal studies.
- Fasting is not a cruel procedure, since (1) mice, as well as humans, can survive with no food for three or four days, and (2) fasting is equally beneficial for them, since it can prevent diseases and help them live longer.

I know that giving chemotherapy to mice makes them suffer. I have issues with that. Nevertheless, I don't see any alternatives if we want to save human lives. For this reason, we limit animal studies to the minimum required, and in general, we target advanced-stage diseases either deadly or devastating to patients.

A few years ago, I responded to a letter from an animal-rights activist with the following question: "If your child, sister, or father was dying, and the only treatment that might save their life needed to be tested first in mice, would you condone the mouse experiments? Or would you choose to see your loved one die?"

I know many activists will still object, but I ask that they be honest and consider the consequences. If they don't condone animal experiments under any circumstances, even those necessary to develop treatments for deadly diseases, then they should never take any drug—even aspirin or antibiotics—and tell their family members to do the same.

I believe animal experiments should be undertaken only as a precursor to human clinical trials in the treatment of advanced-stage and major illnesses. In the absence of better options, these trials are unfortunately a necessary evil.

By winter, Napoleon's army was in tatters after enduring months of starvation, freezing conditions, and the final attack by the Russians. When the war ended, 400,000 of Napoleon's soldiers had perished.

Cancer cells behave like Napoleon's army, advancing even when it would be wiser to stop. To stay alive, they require a lot of nourishment. As stated earlier, the typical nutritional recommendation given by doctors to cancer patients is to "eat normally or more than normal." This makes intuitive sense, as it made intuitive sense for the Russian army to engage Napoleon's invaders the moment they arrived, in the summer of 1812, when they were well fed. Because the Russians waited until the soldiers were at their weakest, the combination of cold, starvation, and targeted attacks by the Russians defeated them permanently. In the same way, starved cancer cells are most vulnerable to the assault of chemotherapy or many other therapies after fasting.

Having conceived the idea of a starvation-induced "magic shield," I remembered a basic lesson from evolutionary biology: the great majority of genetic mutations (changes in the DNA sequence) are deleterious, but their negative consequences usually appear only under certain conditions, like when the environment is particularly hot or cold. As described earlier, mutations in the DNA sequence of cancer cells increase their ability to grow, but those same mutations will greatly impede the cancer cell's ability to survive in challenging environments, for example under the double onslaught of starvation and chemotherapy or immunotherapy.

Could this theoretical scenario actually work? In fact, our mouse studies and those of other researchers show that fasting, in addition to protecting normal cells, makes standard therapy much more toxic to melanoma, breast cancer, prostate cancer, lung cancer, liver cancer, colorectal cancer, neuroblastoma, leukemia, and a number of other cancers. In many cases, cycles of fasting (or of a fasting-mimicking diet) are as effective as chemotherapy at fighting cancer. However, neither strategy alone is optimal. Permanent therapeutic effects are achieved only through the combination of fasting or fasting-mimicking diets and standard cancer therapies developed for a specific cancer. In mouse studies, we saw that fasting combined with various therapies can cure a portion of the mice even in the advanced stages of the disease, after the cancer had metastasized. Not all mice were cured, but we and others regularly obtained a 20 to 60 percent remission rate for a variety of cancers.

I have dedicated different chapters in this book to the description of the effects of fasting and fasting-mimicking diets against various types of cancers, showing both laboratory experiments and, when available, clinical trial results.

FASTING-MIMICKING DIETS AND IMMUNE SYSTEM–DEPENDENT KILLING OF CANCER CELLS

Among new therapies to treat and, in some cases, possibly cure cancer, perhaps the most promising is immunotherapy, which relies on the immune system to kill cancer cells. In another set of very promising animal and clinical studies at USC and in Italy and Spain, we and others showed that fasting or the fasting-mimicking diet can trigger an effect similar to that produced by immunotherapy.[2] Multiple studies, which looked at breast cancer, skin cancer, and lung cancer, found that the fasting-mimicking diet performs four main functions:

1. It weakens cancer cells and the protective shield, making them more easily attacked by the immune system cells.
2. It generates new immune system cells, making the immune system more aggressive toward the cancer.[3]
3. It makes immunotherapy more effective.
4. It reduces the side effects caused by immunotherapy.

The effects of the fasting-mimicking diet on the immune-dependent attack of cancer cells and on making immunotherapy more effective will be discussed in detail in different chapters focusing on specific cancers.

FASTING-MIMICKING DIETS AND CHEMOTHERAPY-RELATED STEROIDS

Corticosteroids (hormones) such as prednisolone, methylprednisolone, and dexamethasone are frequently used in combination with chemotherapy in cancer treatment. In a 2017 publication, we showed that the corticosteroid dexamethasone increased the toxicity of the chemotherapy drug doxorubicin by increasing the level of glucose, i.e., sugar, in the blood of mice.[4]

By increasing the levels of blood glucose, corticosteroids make mice weaker, while seemingly making cancer cells stronger. This effect was reversed by combining dexamethasone and chemotherapy with the fasting-mimicking diet, in part because the fasting period lowered blood glucose levels. Our results indicate that corticosteroids should not be combined with chemotherapy unless there is no viable alternative. In fact, high glucose levels in combination with chemotherapy in patients are associated with an increased risk of developing infections and higher death rates, when compared with patients with normal blood glucose.[5] Thus, both our mouse data and preliminary clinical data indicate that steroid hormones that increase blood glucose levels can be detrimental in combination with chemotherapy.

AN ANTIBIOTIC FOR CANCER? ANTIAGING INTERVENTIONS TO FIGHT CANCER

In September 1928, Alexander Fleming, a Scottish physician and microbiologist, was studying *Staphylococcus*, the bacteria that cause sore throats and other infections. In one petri dish, he noticed that the bacteria were growing everywhere except in an area where mold was growing. Fleming isolated the mold that was toxic to bacteria and identified it as belonging to the *Penicillium* genus; this "mold juice" has become the most widely used antibiotic on the planet. My question, as it is for thousands of doctors and researchers: Is there a penicillin for cancer? What if we can identify medicines that, like penicillin, control or may even cure cancers without causing major side effects to the patient?

My own group has published results that show how certain cancer therapies can be reminiscent of the use of antibiotics against bacteria. Together with Maira Di Tano, a former graduate student in my IFOM laboratory in Milan, we published a study in which we combined two nutrition-related strategies known to protect normal cells from aging—vitamin C and the fasting-mimicking diet—to kill colorectal cancer cells. We already know from many studies in mice and humans that both (especially the fasting-mimicking diet) have protective and antiaging effects. In humans, fasting-mimicking-diet cycles reduce cholesterol, triglycerides, blood pressure, fasting glucose, and other disease risk factors. In mice, fasting-mimicking-diet cycles extend life span and cut cancer incidence nearly in half (see chapter 3 about cancer prevention). But what if the fasting-mimicking diet were combined with another anti-aging nutrient like vitamin C instead of toxic drugs like chemotherapy? I will discuss this in detail in the colorectal cancer chapter. A completely nontoxic intervention including the fasting-mimicking diet, vitamin C, and other nontoxic drugs could eventually generate a cancer medicine more potent than chemotherapy and potentially as effective against cancer as antibiotics are against bacteria; it could be (1) recommended by the doctor when the cancer is diagnosed and (2) utilized for relatively long periods, killing cancer cells without causing damage to the patient.

. . . .

FASTING AS WILD-CARD THERAPY

Because the characteristics of cancer cells[6] are so vast and the current drug therapies can target only one of them at a time, we are in desperate need of a "wild card" therapy that will expand their reach and efficacy. Fasting-mimicking diets act on many of these hallmarks that contribute to cancer survival and growth. One of them in particular—the ability to block cancer cells from rewiring and escaping the toxicity of the treatment—is what makes the fasting-mimicking diet a very promising wild-card therapy. In fact, fasting and fasting-mimicking diets have been shown to do the following in mice, and in initial human clinical studies:

1. Block many escape routes for cancer cells by limiting the availability of nutrients and growth factors.
2. Reduce inflammation.
3. Increase the recognition of different types of tumor cells by the immune system.
4. Trigger cancer cells to ignore orders stopping their growth. (During starvation, conditions stopping growth are an important way for cells to survive; by not stopping growth, cancer cells are more likely to die. Cancer cells are like people who continue to run in the hot desert, despite not having water or any shade.)
5. Promote apoptosis (programmed cell death) by increasing the generation of reactive oxygen molecules that damage cancer cells but also by limiting the factors that stop apoptosis (insulin-like growth factor 1 [IGF-1], etc.), thereby causing cancer cell death.

FASTING AND FASTING-MIMICKING DIETS: STORIES FROM PATIENTS

Since 2008, we have collected a number of anecdotes from cancer patients, some of which I will include at the end of each specific cancer chapter. Many of these patients responded so well to the combination of fasting-mimicking diets and standard therapies that they surprised oncologists. These anecdotes aren't proof that the combination of standard cancer therapy and fasting-mimicking diet cures some cancers, but together with the mouse and clinical data, they point to a potentially effective strategy for improving and in some cases greatly improving conventional treatments while reducing side effects. For example, for several patients in the early stages of some leukemias, the foundation clinics recommended the fasting-mimicking diet and/or the Longevity Diet without drugs, since the standard of care at that stage is "watch and wait," and were able to observe long-term control of the cancer growth.

With the help of doctors Romina Inés Cervigni and Cristina Villa and the foundation clinics teams, as well as my colleagues at various universities, I will present in the following chapters all of the available data for (a) the use of fasting and fasting-mimicking diets in either cancer prevention or the treatment of each type of cancer and (b) the role of the Longevity Diet and other types of everyday nutrition, including the ketogenic diet, that could improve the efficacy of the standard drugs. In many cases, we had available both extensive animal and clinical data, but in others we had only animal data. I have tried to explain the material in a way that is clear to patients, health-care professionals, and oncologists but that also maximizes the safety of patients. For example, in some cases we may have very limited efficacy data for the use of the fasting-mimicking diet in combination with chemotherapy for a specific cancer, but we may have data for clinical research combining it with another cancer type. While this is not the end of the road, it is a great pathway toward the future of curing cancer.

2

GENES, AGING, AND CANCER

GENES THAT CONTROL CANCER

Microorganisms

It was already clear to us in the nineties that the "aging genes" were very effective in accelerating damage and mutations in the DNA and were also very effective in increasing "cancer-like" growth. By deactivating these aging genes with fasting, we drastically reduced both. These genes were the same ones that, when blocked, caused yeast cells to live longer: TOR-Sch9/S6K, which is activated by proteins/amino acids, and RAS-PKA, activated by sugars. The higher levels of amino acids and sugars cause the activation of the TOR-Sch9/S6K and RAS-PKA pathways, which in turn promote growth but accelerate the aging process and DNA damage and mutations, which in mammals can increase the risk of cancer and metastases.

Thus, if these "aging genes" are turned on by sugar and protein, the organism grows in size and also generates more cells. In order to do so, it must take its focus and energy away from protecting the organism against damage, allowing the aging process to proceed at a faster pace for the sake of growth. Producing a newborn organism—a "daughter cell"—makes the damage caused to the DNA and other components of the "mother organism" irrelevant, because the great majority of it will be filtered out during the reproduction process, so that the new daughter organism can have a fresh and youthful start.

Fasting leads to a severe reduction in proteins and sugars, which forces the organism to enter a protected mode, but we discovered it can also act as a filter that cleans and repairs cells and tissues. Because of this self-repair, the organism no longer needs to reproduce. In other words, the fasting and refeeding cycle may represent an ancient opportunity, first evolved in microorganisms billions of years ago and at least partially working in humans, to do the following:

1. remove damaged components, including cancer cells and cellular components;
2. utilize these cancer or damaged cells and cellular components for energy by a cannibalism-like process; and
3. turn on stem cells and reprogram old cells to replace these cancer and other damaged cells with young and functional ones after normal levels of food become again available.

Mice

Yeast are useful for research but ultimately are too simple compared with humans. What about mice? Studies show that reducing the levels of the genes that are activated by proteins and sugars (growth hormone IGF-1, TOR-S6K, insulin, and PKA) can cause the mice not only to live longer but remarkably also to show a major reduction in tumors.

In one study, the causes of death were compared for two groups of forty-five mice. In the first group, the mice had very low levels of growth factors (which are also reduced during fasting and protein restriction), and the second group were normal mice. Results revealed that while 87 percent of normal mice died of tumors, only 40 percent of the mice that had very low levels of growth factors died of tumors, with a major reduction in the incidence of lymphomas and breast cancer.[1] Similarly, in another long-lived group of mice that had low levels of growth factors, 42 percent died from tumors, compared with 83 percent of the normal mice.[2]

This showed that the mice with low levels of growth factors can have a major reduction in tumor incidence compared to normal mice. As importantly, growth factors–deficient mice live about 40 percent longer. In fact, if we consider the 40 percent longer life span, the average monthly tumor number is reduced about three-fold in mice with severe growth-factors reduction.[3]

In addition to cancer prevention, cancer progression in mice with low growth factors is often slower than cancer progression in normal mice (figure 2.1). This suggests that these genes are controlling not only whether the mice get cancer or not but also how the tumors survive and grow after they are formed.

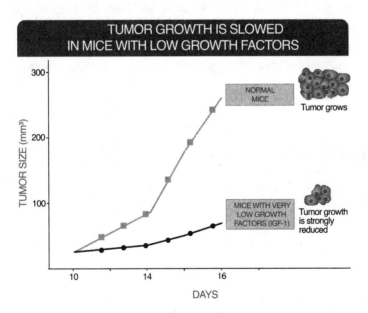

2.1. *Tumor progression of melanoma in mice with a growth hormone receptor (GHR) deficiency and with low levels of growth factors (insulin-like growth factor 1, IGF-1) is strongly inhibited compared with progression in normal mice. This helps us to understand that the growth hormone receptor (GHR) and IGF-1 can promote not only tumor formation but also its progression.*

These experiments were repeated and confirmed by multiple laboratories with different types of yeast and mice. These results indicate that the effects of growth genes on DNA damage or cancer incidence are likely to be similar for single-celled organisms, mice, and even humans.

Humans

In 2003, I wrote a review for *Science* magazine entitled "Evolutionary Medicine: From Dwarf Model Systems to Healthy Centenarians?" with Caleb Finch of the University of Southern California. In it, we proposed a new approach that could change the way we think about medicine, focusing much more on the nutrition and genes that can extend healthy longevity rather than on drugs that delay disease progression. Mice and humans are both mammals, yet one is able to prevent cancer for a thirty-times-longer period than the other, based on the evolution of a much more sophisticated anti-aging and anti-cancer program. I called it "evolutionary medicine" and used this picture in the article to illustrate that fact (figure 2.2):

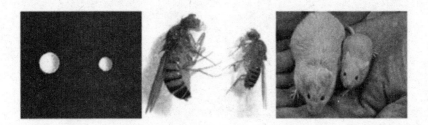

2.2. *Yeast, flies, and mice. On the left of each picture is the organism without mutations in growth genes. On the right is the organism with mutations impairing growth. These mutations are important to live longer: Mutated dwarf yeast (right) survives three times longer than normal yeast (left), and its DNA is protected. Dwarf flies (right) can live twice as long as normal flies (left). Dwarf mice (right) show a life span extension of 40 percent compared to normal mice (left), and the number of their tumors is halved. Valter D. Longo and Caleb E. Finch, "Evolutionary Medicine: From Dwarf Model Systems to Heathy Centenarians?,"* Science 299, no. 5611 (2003): 1342–46.

The article also features a graph from a study by Richard Miller entitled "Extending Life: Scientific Prospects and Political Obstacles." This graph (figure 2.3) shows why treating aging can potentially achieve a bigger bang for the buck compared with treating diseases and that investing in aging research would provide many more years of healthy lives than even cures for cancer, heart disease, stroke, and diabetes *combined*. This is not an attempt to minimize the importance of research on specific diseases, but it does point to the need to complement it with a major focus on research on aging and healthy longevity.

With the theory of evolutionary medicine in place, in 2003 I

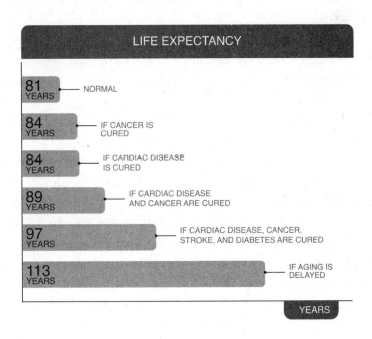

2.3. *In 1985, life expectancy was eighty-one years. Starting from this information, the authors of this study calculated how much longer we would live if illnesses like cancer (84 years), cardiac disease (84 years), cancer and cardiac disease (89 years), or cancer, cardiac disease, stroke, and diabetes (97 years) disappeared. The authors suggest that by delaying aging, as demonstrated in mice and many other organisms, we hypothetically could live for 113 years on average. Modified from Richard A. Miller, "Extending Life: Scientific Prospects and Political Obstacles," Milbank Quarterly 80, no. 1 (March 2002): 155–74.*

started to redirect my attention from dwarf yeast, flies, and mice to humans. I wondered, were there people with deficiencies in growth hormone or the growth-hormone receptor just like the long-lived mice protected from cancer? I wrote to Zvi Laron, a pediatric endocrinologist in Israel who discovered and named Laron syndrome in humans, which is caused by a mutation in the same growth hormone receptor gene that makes mice small and long-lived (figure 2.2). Laron pointed me to a very old group of people on the island of Krk in Croatia who had deficiency in the growth hormone receptor (Laron syndrome) and who lived into their nineties without cancer or other diseases. These were fascinating cases, but they were not going to be enough to determine whether the growth hormone receptor gene also protected humans from aging and diseases.

Luckily, around 2004, I had shared my theory with Hassy Cohen, who at the time was the chief of pediatric endocrinology at UCLA. He listened to my idea and told me, "You know who follows many people who have that exact mutation? His name is Jaime Guevara-Aguirre, a pediatric endocrinologist who for many years has been studying the growth defects in children in the Andes mountains of southern Ecuador with mutations in the growth hormone receptor gene, also called GHRD or Laron syndrome." I could not believe it. This was perfect. Within a few hours I had already written to Dr. Guevara, and within a few months I invited him to present at a conference in Los Angeles. The results he first presented were not about aging and disease, since he had focused on children's growth, but he did tell me that he did not remember seeing cancer in the GHRD group. In 2005, I visited them and the two things that struck me were (1) they had a terrible diet, and (2) they were always happy, and loved joking and laughing (figure 2.4).

I thought the time necessary to determine whether this Ecuadorian group was protected from cancer would be relatively brief. That was not the case. It took us six years to have a convincing enough case to publish our work in *Science Translational Medicine*.[4]

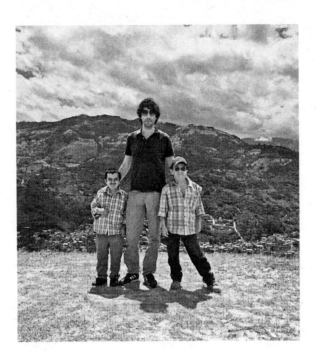

2.4. *In Ecuador with two people with Laron syndrome, characterized by low levels of growth factors, which causes short height. However, the same genetic defect protects many such people from many diseases (including cancer and diabetes), despite an unhealthy lifestyle and diet.*

Our conclusions were:

1. GHRD people with very low growth factors were protected from cancer. In the thirty years that Jaime Guevara followed them, only one person had died of cancer. Zvi Laron had published similar results for people with GHRD mutations in the Middle East and Europe (figure 2.5).[5]

2. Even though GHRD people followed an unhealthy diet, did not exercise, and were usually more overweight and obese than their normal relatives, they rarely developed diabetes or insulin resistance, which precedes diabetes. They also had normal glucose levels. This second finding is important for cancer, since both high levels of insulin and high levels of glucose can accelerate aging and

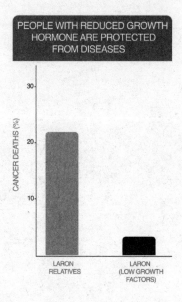

PEOPLE WITH REDUCED GROWTH
HORMONE ARE PROTECTED
FROM DISEASES

2.5. *People with a deficiency of the growth hormone receptor at birth have a short stature and have a much lower chance of dying of cancer than other members of their families who live in the same house and eat the same food. Modified from Jaime Guevara-Aguirre et al., "Growth Hormone Receptor Deficiency Is Associated with a Major Reduction in Pro-Aging Signaling, Cancer, and Diabetes in Humans," Science Translational Medicine, 3, no. 7 (2011): 70ra13.*

cancer development, as well as help cancer cells survive and grow. As you will read later, insulin and glucose levels, which are low in GHRD and high in diabetic patients, can play key roles in increasing cancer incidence and progression.

We knew that the scientific journals would not believe our conclusions unless we also demonstrated this at the cellular and molecular level. For this reason, before we submitted the study for publication, we took human epithelial cells (those that give rise to breast, prostate, and many other cancers) and exposed them to a cancer-causing agent using either blood from GHRD people or blood from their relatives. We obtained both expected and surprising results:

A. The DNA damage was much lower in the epithelial cells that were exposed to carcinogens and the GHRD blood. This was the expected finding.

B. The epithelial cells incubated in GHRD blood and damaged by carcinogens died much more rapidly than those incubated in the normal blood. We did not expect this, but we should have, since IGF-1 has been well established to block the suicide of cells (including cancer cells) that are damaged.

In other words, the people with GHRD were doubly protected: first by reducing the DNA damage caused by the carcinogen, then by increasing the suicide and removal of cells that became

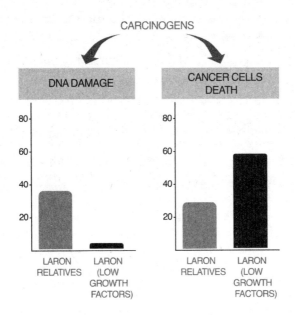

2.6. *In this experiment, epithelial cells, the type that can give rise to many types of cancers, were mixed with a substance that favors the development of tumors (carcinogen). Cells behaved differently depending on whether they were exposed to normal blood (from normal relatives of Laron people, on the left of each graph) or blood with low levels of growth hormones (from Laron people, on the right of each graph). Cells exposed to normal blood had more DNA damage and were protected from cell death/suicide. Modified from Guevara-Aguirre et al.,* Science Translational Medicine, *2011.*

damaged and could proceed to become cancer cells, thanks in part to the very low concentration of the growth factor IGF-1 in their blood (figure 2.6).

In a later publication[6] we demonstrated that reductions of IGF-1 played a key role in the effects of fasting and the fasting-mimicking diet in the treatment of mice with breast cancer receiving hormone therapy, thus providing a connection between the role of genetics and growth hormone receptor deficiency and that of nutrition and fasting in cancer prevention and treatment (see also chapter 3).

THIS RESEARCH ON GENES AND their very potent effect on cancer points to a shift in how we should think about the disease. These findings suggest that it is now possible to create drugs that delay aging and also use them for cancer prevention—but to move this concept from the laboratory to the clinic could take decades. Until then, but probably also after that, nutrition and fasting-mimicking-diet cycles—which can control the levels of insulin and IGF-1 as well as glucose, leptin (a hormone produced by fat cells that assists in the regulation of fat storage and regulates glucose levels), and many other factors that promote aging—can provide perhaps the most potent tool in cancer prevention and possibly a game-changing tool in cancer treatment.

3

FASTING, NUTRITION, AND PHYSICAL ACTIVITY IN CANCER PREVENTION

For their contributions to this chapter and its revision, I would like to thank Mario Mirisola, PhD, associate professor of applied dietary technical sciences in the Department of Oncological and Gastric Surgical Disciplines at the University of Palermo; Annalisa Arrighi, PhD, osteopath; and Romina Inés Cervigni, PhD, chief scientific officer of Fondazione Valter Longo in Milan and the Create Cures Foundation in Los Angeles.

FASTING AND NUTRITION

When asked if fasting is good or bad for health, I often say that "fasting" doesn't mean anything, since it can refer to a period without food consumption lasting from a few hours to a few months, which could be done once a day or once a year. It is like asking if eating is good for your health. The answer is that both eating and fasting are good, bad, and neutral for your health and longevity, but they can be very beneficial if done correctly and appropriately for the right person at the right time and frequency. The purpose of this chapter is to identify the best and most feasible forms of fasting and to show how powerful they can be against cancer. I will also briefly discuss the types of fasting that can be both good and those that appear to be unhealthy. I suggest that you speak to one of our foundation's nutrition professionals or doctors to receive further guidance.

Many articles have been written on the benefits of fasting, and the practice has been part of human history starting thousands of years ago. Some religions use fasting as a form of ritual and sacrifice. But just because something has been adopted for thousands of years does not necessarily mean it is good for your health. For example, for centuries, family elders recommended to eat as much as possible in order to prevent malnourishment. But now that practice is responsible for over 70 percent of Americans and around 60 percent of Europeans being overweight or obese. But as described in my book *The Longevity Diet*, eating a lot can be a solution and not a problem; as long as the food is low-sugar, vegan, or pescatarian, it has high volume and fiber but relatively low-calorie content, allowing a person to maintain a normal weight. There is much complexity to nutrition and its links to cells, genes, and cancer. Thus, it is important to understand how and why fasting was utilized for thousands of years, but it is more important to identify the type of fasting that works best to live long and cancer free or to treat cancer based on the science.

TIME-RESTRICTED EATING AND THE FASTING-MIMICKING DIET IN CANCER PREVENTION

When it comes to the number of hours in which to fast, many factors come into play depending on desired outcomes, and there are potentially different effects caused by different lengths and starting times. In a sixteen-week trial, people who fasted for a fourteen-hour window (eating within a ten-hour range each day) showed a reduction in body weight, maintained after one year.[1] They also saw improved energy in the morning and throughout the day, reduced hunger at bedtime, and improved sleep.

Fasting periods longer than thirteen hours (fourteen to twenty hours), however, have been shown to be problematic. For example, people who skip breakfast and who may be fasting daily for sixteen hours or more show higher LDL, diabetes, and heart disease, as well as increased mortality.[2] Long fasting periods also increase the risk of developing gallstones: sixteen hours of daily fasting carries double the chance of hospitalization with gallstone-related symptoms compared with ten hours or less of daily fasting, possibly because longer fasting promotes the accumulation of high levels of cholesterol in the bile.[3] Therefore daily fasting periods longer than thirteen hours are not advised for the generally healthy population.

Thus, a good compromise to reap the benefits of intermittent fasting while reducing health risks may be twelve to thirteen hours of daily/nightly fasting. A particularly interesting clinical study was conducted by Satchin Panda, one of the pioneers of time-restricted eating and a professor at the Salk Institute in San Diego. Through a mobile app, he monitored how eating for fifteen hours or more can negatively affect weight, sleep, and energy levels.[4] When food consumption was limited to fewer than eleven hours during the day, beneficial effects on weight, sleep, and energy levels were observed.

BASED ON THIS EVIDENCE, MY recommendation for relatively healthy people, as described in *The Longevity Diet*, is generally consistent with the work of Satchin Panda: eat for eleven to twelve hours per day and then fast for twelve to thirteen hours a night. I have yet to see a negative study associated with a twelve-hour fast, suggesting that if it does cause problems, they are rare.

With regard to cancer, overnight fasting has been shown to

improve the regulation of blood glucose and sleep, and these factors potentially reduce the risk of cancer recurrence. For example, in 2016[5] a study found that nightly fasting duration of thirteen hours or fewer per night is associated with a higher chance for breast cancer recurrence (36 percent) compared with fasting thirteen or more hours per night, in a group of women taking part in the prospective Women's Healthy Eating and Living study between 1995 and 2007. Based on this recent evidence, women with familial risk of breast cancer, or even those already affected by this kind of cancer, may want to consider nightly fasting of thirteen to fourteen hours. For example, someone could finish dinner by 7:00 p.m. and begin breakfast between 8:00 and 9:00 a.m.

Maintaining an adequate daily fasting period of thirteen to fourteen hours represents a simple and feasible way to potentially reduce breast cancer recurrence without also potentially increasing side effects like gallstones or cardiovascular disease. The reason for this effect may be that fasting lowers the average levels of blood glucose, insulin, and leptin and reduces abdominal fat, IGF-1, and other growth factors, all of which are associated with cancer progression in either animal or human studies. This has multiple benefits, as it also helps reduce the risk of type 2 diabetes and cardiovascular disease.

IN ADDITION TO THE TWELVE- to thirteen-hour daily fasting period (in healthy people), my laboratory and a range of hospitals that we collaborate with have published data indicating that fasting-mimicking-diet cycles carried out once a month to once every three or four months cause improvements associated with delayed aging and disease prevention. Five-day fasting-mimicking diets, which are plant-based, low calorie, low protein, low sugar, and high fat, have been shown in multiple clinical trials to reduce potential risk factors and markers for cancer, including IGF-1, insulin, leptin, and glucose, as well as abdominal fat and waist circumference.[6]

· · · · · · ·

CALORIE RESTRICTION

For more than a hundred years we have known that reducing calorie intake by 20 to 40 percent below a normal intake (known as calorie restriction or CR) not only causes mice to live longer but also reduces and postpones different types of cancers. Although many have heard about the remarkable effects of calorie restriction, fewer people know that when mice of different genetic backgrounds are tested, calorie restriction increases life span in about a third of the mice, it has no effect in another third, and it shortens the life spans of the final third. This indicates that chronic calorie restriction can be good, neutral, or bad depending on the genetic background of the mouse, although it is too early to know whether this range of effects is also observed in humans.

In one study, calorie restriction without changes in the type of food consumed reduced cancer by 50 percent in monkeys, but in another study its effects were much smaller.[7] However, this research demonstrates that many cancers can be prevented by chronic calorie restriction, but because it is very difficult to follow and it is accompanied by severe weight and muscle loss, it is not feasible for most people.

Our studies show that Ecuadorian people with a mutation in the growth hormone receptor gene rarely develop cancer, which is in agreement with similar findings for people with the same mutation in Europe and the Middle East, even though these populations represent many different genetic backgrounds. As described earlier, similar results were obtained in mice with mutations in the same growth genes, which are protected from cancer but also live 40 percent longer. Together, these studies indicate that many and possibly most cancers can be prevented by dietary restrictions affecting growth genes but also suggest that these dietary interventions cannot include chronic calorie restriction, since they must be feasible and cause minimal or no side effects. The goal for these dietary and other lifestyle interventions should not be just to prevent a single disease, like cancer, but to delay aging to prevent many diseases. However, I do want to touch on cancer prevention specifically, especially for those who have a genetic predisposition to cancer (many cancers in the family) and also those who are exposed to environments that promote cancer (toxins in food, pollution, etc.). For them, the two lines of defense are (1) diets and exercise that regulate the genes that control aging and cancer, and (2) limiting exposure to agents that can cause or increase cancer (carcinogens, growth hormones, viruses, etc.).

HEREDITARY CANCER

Cancer can be caused by carcinogenic substances that damage DNA, such as tobacco, pollution, and radiation, and/or by lifestyle factors, such as obesity and poor nutrition. However, about 5 to 10 percent of all cancers may be caused by the genes we inherit from our parents, specifically genes with mutations that can increase the risk of cancer. For more than fifty hereditary cancer types, mutations predispose individuals to developing that cancer.

For example, people with defects in the alcohol dehydrogenase (ADH) enzyme have trouble metabolizing alcohol, which can increase the risk of pancreatic cancer. This genetic defect is very common in some populations, such as the Japanese and other Eastern Asian ethnicities,[8] and those with it should avoid drinking alcohol. These predispositions require specific preventive changes, but the majority of people can also likely benefit from a genetic-specific diet that includes various food sources that were eaten by their ancestors (for example, chickpeas for those of southern European ancestry and soybeans for those of Asian ancestry). In the following section, I discuss how different types of fasting and everyday nutrition can affect cancer incidence, which can help those with a predisposition to the disease.

. . . . . .

AGING AND CANCER PREVENTION

Cancer is perhaps the most representative age-related disease, primarily because it depends on a group of factors strongly affected by the aging process, including DNA damage, inflammation, and reduced function of the immune system. Therefore, the prevention of cancer is more in line with the delay of the aging process and the activation of anti-aging systems compared to many other diseases. A slightly modified version of the Longevity Diet is the focus of this cancer prevention chapter. In my previous book,[9] I discuss the Five Pillars of Longevity, which combine different fields of science and medicine to provide dietary and other lifestyle recommendations highly likely to improve health and extend life. The purpose of the pillars (described in *The Longevity Diet*) is to move away from any single study or even field of research (such as epidemiological studies) to recommendations that are supported by all or the great majority of the different pillars—that are unlikely to undergo major changes in the next few decades, based on new studies being published.[10]

JUVENTOLOGY RESEARCH

I coined the term *juventology* to provide an alternative to the idea of studying the aging process (gerontology) and to focus instead on studying the youth period (youth span) and how to maintain it and even partially return to it. Why does a mouse get cancer at middle age (around eighteen months of age), while humans are rarely diagnosed with cancer before thirty to forty years of age? The answer is that mice and humans are controlled by two very different longevity programs regulated by different DNA sequences. The mouse program makes sure that it stays young and free of cancer for a little over one year, while the human one ensures that the great majority of people remain functional and cancer free until the end of their prime reproductive years (thirty to forty years of age). This tells us that (1) no matter which program is activated, cancer is not unavoidable, and (2) by delaying aging we can also delay, and in many cases avoid, cancer.

THE LONGEVITY DIET AND CANCER PREVENTION

In my first book, I detail the Longevity Diet—a heavily researched nutritional program to slow down cellular aging and reduce the risk of the onset of cardiovascular and autoimmune diseases, diabetes, and neurodegenerative diseases such as Alzheimer's—and cancer. Based on the Five Pillars of Longevity, the plan's main guidelines are below (and I recommend reading the book if you decide to follow the program):[11]

1. Eat mostly (but not exclusively) vegan, avoiding animal products as much as possible but consuming fish two or three times a week. Choose fish with high omega-3, omega-6, and vitamin B12 content (salmon, anchovies, sardines, cod, sea bream, trout, clams, and shrimp). It is important to buy high-quality fish and choose those with low levels of mercury.

2. If you are younger than sixty-five, keep protein intake low (0.8 grams of protein per kilogram of body weight or 0.36 grams per pound of body weight). This means 47 grams of protein per day for a person weighing 59 kilos (130 pounds) and 80 grams of protein per day for someone weighing 100 kilos (220 pounds). Consume a balance of black beans, chickpeas, green peas, lentils, and other legumes as well as oilseeds (pumpkin seeds, sesame, linseeds, etc.), nuts (walnuts, almonds, hazelnuts, etc.), and low-mercury fish as your main sources of protein. If your main source of proteins is legumes, increase protein intake by 10 to 20 percent. Above the age of sixty-five, you should increase protein intake by 20 percent, adding

more fish, eggs, white meat, and products from goats and sheep to preserve muscle mass and increase nourishment.[12] In this age range legumes should not provide the majority of the protein consumed.

3. Minimize saturated fats from animal sources (meat and cheese) and plant sources as well as sugar and starch-rich food (pasta, bread, rice, potatoes, etc.) while maximizing plant-based, unsaturated fats and complex carbs. Eat whole grains and high quantities of vegetables (tomatoes, broccoli, carrots, legumes, etc.) together with olive oil (three tablespoons per day) and nuts (1 ounce [28 grams] per day),[13] always being mindful of intolerances and allergies (for instance, tomatoes, nuts, eggplant, etc.), and prevent unwanted weight gain.

4. Follow a diet with high vitamin and mineral content, supplemented with a multivitamin. Theoretically a diet rich in vegetables, fish, nuts, and whole grains plus fruit is the ideal way to get all the nutrients you need, but most people have deficiencies and supplementation may be helpful. My recommendation is to take a multivitamin that is produced by a reputable company and contains at least vitamin A, vitamin D, vitamin E, magnesium, calcium, potassium, and vitamin K. Take the supplement every two to three days to minimize the chance of a toxic effect.

5. Among the healthy ingredients listed above, select mostly those that your ancestors would have eaten frequently.

6. Based on your weight, age, and abdominal circumference, decide whether to have two or three meals per day. If you are overweight or tend to gain weight easily, consume two meals a day: breakfast and either lunch or dinner, plus one low-sugar (less than five grams of sugar or starch) snack with fewer than one hundred calories. If you are already at a normal weight, or if you tend to lose weight easily or are over sixty-five and of normal weight,

       eat three meals a day plus one low-sugar/low-starch snack with fewer than one hundred calories.

7. Confine all eating to a twelve-hour period; for example, start at 8:00 a.m. and end at 8:00 p.m. Don't eat anything within three to four hours of bedtime.

8. Consider between two and twelve five-day-long fasting-mimicking diets per year depending on your needs (for example, two fasting-mimicking diets per year if you are in good shape, have low BMI, and are healthy, twelve fasting-mimicking diets during year one—under a doctor's supervision—if you are diabetic).

9. Buy organic food[14] with no pesticides[15] or antibiotics[16] when you can. Use oral antibiotics only when necessary.

10. Drink a maximum of two to three glasses of (preferably red) wine or beer per week (and only if you are not at risk for certain cancers).[17]

11. Make sure to exercise. (The following section is dedicated to physical activity that helps prevent cancers.)

PHYSICAL ACTIVITY IN CANCER PREVENTION AND TREATMENT

FOR THEIR CONTRIBUTIONS IN WRITING this section, I thank Annalisa Arrighi, PhD, osteopath, and Romina Inés Cervigni, PhD, scientific director of Fondazione Valter Longo in Milan; for the contribution and revision, I thank Massimo Lanza, PhD, associate professor of methods for teaching physical education and sports at the Department of Neuroscience, Biomedicine, and Movement at the University of Verona.

WHEN WE EXERCISE, WE SHOULD do enough to help our overall health but not overdo it to the point where we injure ourselves. When done correctly, exercise can promote important changes in almost all systems of the human body responsible for regulating cellular aging, damage to DNA, and the survival and growth of cancer cells.[18]

To improve health and counter the development of cancer, both aerobic and anaerobic activity are required. The term *aerobic* refers to a type of metabolism in which cells rely on oxygen and glucose (sugar) in order to produce energy. More strenuous aerobic activity usually results in greater benefit to our system. When the intensity (and therefore the effort) of the exercise increases significantly, cellular metabolism no longer remains mostly aerobic but becomes predominantly anaerobic: the cell no longer receives sufficient oxygen and therefore turns to other metabolic pathways in order to produce energy, mostly through the use of glycogen, our carbohydrate reserve that forms in the liver. Both aerobic exercises, such as walking, running, or riding a bicycle, and short, fast, and high-intensity anaerobic exercises used to develop and maintain muscle strength are needed, in particular after age forty, when there is a significant reduction of muscle mass and strength.

This section will illustrate how to optimize longevity and help prevent tumors through physical exercise and, subsequently, describe state-of-the-art physical activity focusing on both exercises aimed at cancer prevention and those to be used during cancer therapy, with the aim of setting an ideal "amount" for each individual.

How to Optimize Longevity and Cancer Prevention Through Exercise and Physical Activity

We know that physical activity reduces the risk of cancer, but studies also show the reverse association between physical activity and the frequency of cancer in a given population. Epidemiological data obtained from seventy-three studies conducted in many countries indicate a 25 percent reduction of breast cancer risk in women who are more physically active compared with those who are less active.[19] Numerous other studies have shown evidence for the protective role physical activity has in reducing many other types of cancer, such as lung, endometrial, colon, kidney, and prostate cancers.[20]

A recent study on almost fifteen thousand British men and women between the ages of forty and seventy-nine indicated that being consistently physically active in middle age provides a substantial health benefit.[21] Researchers have found that transitioning from a sedentary lifestyle to moderate physical activity for at least 150 minutes a week—the minimum amount of physical activity suggested by the World Health Organization—leads to a 24 percent reduction of mortality risk and an 11 percent reduction of the mortality risk linked to cancer. All participants benefited from the physical activity, even those who already suffered from a severe chronic condition, suggesting that at least moderate physical activity acts on both aging and cancer.

Increasing exercise and reducing sedentary behavior, along with increasing occupational and recreational physical activity, may also be a useful strategy to prevent cancer, especially colon cancer.[22] An interesting study published in *Cancer* in 2019 by a team of researchers at the Johns Hopkins School of Medicine in Baltimore demonstrated that individuals who were highly physically active presented a significantly lower risk of developing lung cancer or colorectal cancer compared with those who led a sedentary lifestyle: respectively 77 percent less for lung cancer and 61 percent less for colorectal cancer. Moreover, among the people who developed lung cancer, those who were physically active had a 44 percent lower risk of mortality. Among those affected by colorectal cancer, the probability of death was 89 percent lower when patients were physically active.[23] Notably, these numbers may be affected by selection bias, that is, by selecting cancer patients who exercise because they are healthier or responding better to therapy or more determined to beat the cancer, which would explain the 89 percent lower death risk. Nonetheless, it is clearly important to exercise, and it is likely that a significant portion of these effects are in fact due to the exercise and not to the selection of healthier individuals. Below is a list of the most recent international exercise guidelines for healthy longevity.

Keeping Active

First, everyone should try to walk or bike to work and around town to complete daily tasks. In addition to this activity for at least one hour per day, the recommendation is to do at least 150 minutes of aerobic exercise of moderate intensity (fewer than 25 minutes a day) or 75 minutes of more intense exercise a week.

An aerobic exercise is considered to be of moderate intensity when (1) it causes a slight increase in the heartbeat and respiratory rate and (2) you are still able to talk but unable to sing. When doing a high-intensity exercise, on the other hand, even talking will be difficult. The intensity can be evaluated by measuring the heartbeat. The 150 minutes can be broken up as desired, but I recommend 45 minutes every other day. Again, in addition to these 150 minutes of weekly exercise I recommend one hour a day of walking. In the walking category, only fast walking should be included in the moderate-intensity aerobic exercise portion of the 150 minutes.

There are countless aerobic exercises, and fast walking is probably the most common, but valid alternatives are running, swimming, or using an exercise bike at home when going outdoors isn't an option. Activities such as commuting by bicycle or on foot and hobbies such as gardening or physical labor, even doing daily chores, all contribute to aerobic exercise, but they can be included in either the one hour a day of activity or the 150 minutes of exercise, although at least 10 percent of the 150 minutes should be in the form of more vigorous exercise (jogging, uphill biking, stairs, etc.).

Summary

1. Avoid being sedentary for more than an hour. Interrupt long periods of sitting with a few minutes of physical activity.
2. Take the stairs instead of escalators and elevators.

3. Practice at least 150 minutes of moderate physical activity with at least 15 minutes of vigorous physical activity per week; or 75 minutes of vigorous physical activity per week.

4. Organize training sessions that include weight lifting and stretching for joint mobility twice a week.[24]

5. Go for long walks, avoiding polluted areas if possible. Try to walk at least one hour per day.

6. To maximize muscle growth, consume at least thirty grams of protein in a single meal one to two hours after a relatively intense weight-training session two to three times a week.[25]

7. Drink an adequate amount of water based on your physical activity level and consume sufficient minerals.

Physical Activity and Cancer Treatment

Physical activity can play a major role in patients who are undergoing cancer treatments: it can improve the effectiveness of drugs, reduce side effects, and reduce the risk of developing other pathologies (figure 3.1).[26]

The precise effects of physical exercise on cancer are unclear, but they are likely partially related to weight loss, which helps reduce glucose and insulin levels. A randomized study examined the

PHYSICAL EXERCISE

| CANCER PREVENTION | POSITIVE EFFECT ON ANTITUMORAL THERAPY | REDUCED LONG-TERM SIDE EFFECTS | REDUCED DEVELOPMENT OF METASTASES |

3.1. *Physical activity is important (1) for cancer prevention; (2) during therapy in order to obtain greater tolerance to the drugs and possibly increase their efficacy; (3) to prevent muscle loss and frailty during treatment and after treatment has ended; and (4) to possibly help prevent metastases and as a way to reduce the risk of developing other pathologies. Modified from Pernille Hojman et al., "Molecular Mechanisms Linking Exercise to Cancer Prevention and Treatment,"* Cell Metabolism *27, no. 1 (2018): 10–21.*

effects of different physical-activity interventions on insulin, IGF-1, and adiponectin (a hormone produced by the adipose tissue) on a total of 618 patients taken from eighteen different studies. It concluded that physical activity reduces only insulin levels, not glucose levels, indicating that it may have limited efficacy in improving the treatment of cancers sensitive to glucose levels.[27]

Physical Activity as a Preparation for Surgery

Research published in 2020[28] points to a growing awareness of the difficult but important period between a diagnosis of cancer and the beginning of therapy or surgery. More and more view this time as a crucial moment of preparation. This "pre-habilitation" can help prepare people for treatment by optimizing their physical and mental well-being through exercise, diet, and psychological support. An intervention that includes adequate physical activity can also improve the effectiveness of the treatment and cancer survival rate. Pre-habilitation also helps patients feel a sense of control over their own resources and motivation. In patients with lung cancer, studies have shown that physical activity reduces the post-operation complications and the duration of the recovery period in the hospital. Moreover, adequate physical activity pre-operation can make patients who were previously deemed inoperable eligible for surgery.[29]

Physical Activity and Exercise for Cancer Patients

In the past, physical activity was not considered to be important during cancer treatment. The prevailing idea was (and still is for many hospitals and centers) that cancer patients undergoing chemotherapy and other therapies should avoid any type of exertion.

However, in 1989, a randomized study of forty-five women undergoing adjuvant chemotherapy (therapy subsequent to a surgical operation) for stage II breast cancer (in which the cancer cells have spread only to the breast or nearby lymph nodes) showed that ten

weeks of aerobic activity not only improved their ability to perform tasks that required physical effort but also reduced nausea
induced by chemotherapy. This pioneering work proved that aerobic activity was feasible, safe, and advantageous for patients undergoing chemotherapy.[30]

Since then, studies have accurately documented the positive effects of physical activity in patients undergoing chemotherapy or
radiation therapy for different types of cancer.[31] Physical activity
can ease the side effects of chemotherapy and radiation, including
fatigue and nausea, and can also accelerate recovery from surgery
and the effects of radiation, improving the patient's quality of life.

Physical activity should be continued after treatment ends to
also reduce the chance of cancer recurrence. I recommend working with a cancer exercise specialist or someone well versed in exercise in cancer patients, if possible. It is best to begin gradually
and continue physical activity even in patients who may find it
difficult because of fatigue or other therapy side effects. In fact,
studies have shown that any physical activity is better than none,
whereas stopping physical activity for long periods of time re-
verses any benefit gained and is debilitating overall.[32]

With the help of these studies, the idea that physical activity
can reduce the side effects of cancer treatment and aid in recovery
and rehabilitation after treatment has gained substantial ground.
Observational studies in patients who have overcome breast cancer, colon cancer, and prostate cancer have shown concrete links
between the patient's level of activity and a reduction of the risk
of mortality for their specific cancer type. Moreover, cancer survivors who increase their level of physical activity reduce their all-
cause mortality risk.

The quantity and intensity of exercise needed to register a
benefit in life expectancy appear to vary based on the type of tumor. For example, a reduction of the mortality risk linked to breast
cancer is observed with exercise equivalent to three hours of walking per week; for colon cancer instead, six hours a week shows the
most benefit.[33]

Even in advanced stages of cancer, where the patient may be physically impaired, a moderate type of exercise can help with recovery. It can also improve sexual dysfunction in men undergoing androgen-deprivation therapy in cases of advanced prostate cancer.[34]

Combining Nutrition and Exercise: The Clinical Study in Genoa

In 2020, at the San Martino Hospital in Genoa, Italy, we conducted a clinical study that included a section focused on muscle training in collaboration with Professor Alessio Nencioni's group and oncologists from several hospitals.[35] For the duration of the study, patients received instructions regarding what diet to follow during a five-day cycle of the fasting-mimicking diet once a month. The goal was to follow the amount of protein (mainly from legumes and fish), essential fatty acids, vitamins, and minerals recommended by international guidelines. Patients were also encouraged to partake in strength training daily in a light to moderate form (for twenty minutes). We monitored muscle function and muscle mass (fat mass and lean mass).[36]

Patients were encouraged to follow a routine created by Dr. Annalisa Arrighi, which included exercises to perform at least three or four times a week for a duration of thirty to forty minutes per session (ideally one to two hours before a main meal). (You can find these exercises on the Create Cures website.)

The exercises were simple and had been studied specifically to stimulate the active mobilization of the torso and upper and lower limbs. They included postural and stretching exercises, as well as activities targeting the legs and arms. The study showed that patients who followed our nutritional and training instructions maintained a stable body weight and handgrip strength (a reliable measure of upper-limb strength). The study also indicated that after many cycles of hormone therapy for breast cancer, patients' markers for muscle function and mass increased while fat mass diminished when these cycles were paired with muscle training and a fasting-mimicking diet followed by a diet with normal calories and proteins.[37] It is important to balance the effect of calories and proteins on muscle with their effects on cancer cells, as high levels of nutrients and particularly sugars and proteins could accelerate cancer growth and protect cancer cells from death.

Based on current knowledge, I firmly believe that physical activity can be considered an integral part of cancer treatment, but it should be prescribed by a doctor in tandem with conventional cancer therapy. An assessment of the individual patient's physical condition should be used to determine the recommendations for the initial physical activity and for an adequate progression of its intensity.

In Summary: Optimizing Cancer Treatment and Recovery Through Exercise

An important block of research from the American College of Sports Medicine, the American Cancer Society, and fifteen other organizations has been extracted and condensed into guidelines for people living with cancer.[38] Here is a summary of those guidelines:

- Always consult your doctor or health-care professional to ensure the exercises are appropriate for your specific condition.
- Be physically active both before and after periods of therapy; it is advisable and safe.
- Resume normal activities as soon as possible after treatment.
- Avoid inactivity or sedentary periods.
- Gradually reach the recommended level of physical activity. Try to be consistently physically active over time.
- Work out for the minimum-level recommendation of 90 minutes of moderate aerobic activity (walking, running, cycling, dancing, etc.) per week. Alternatively, 45 minutes a week of high-intensity aerobic activity or even a combi-

nation of moderate and vigorous activity (for example, 60 minutes of moderate activity with 15 minutes of vigorous activity) can be performed by patients who are healthy and strong enough.

- Try to do additional activities or exercises targeting strength and flexibility at least twice a week.

- Consult with your doctor on the type of physical activity best suited to you, particularly in cases of impediment caused by therapy or in the presence of a catheter.

4

FASTING, NUTRITION, AND BREAST CANCER

For their contributions and revisions to this chapter, I thank Debasish Tripathy, MD, chairman of breast medical oncology at the University of Texas MD Anderson Cancer Center in Houston; Giuseppe Curigliano, MD, head of the Division of Early Drug Development at the European Institute of Oncology, IRCCS, in Milan, and associate professor of medical oncology at the University of Milan; Alessandro Laviano, MD, associate professor of medicine in the Department of Translational and Precision Medicine at Sapienza University of Rome; Andreas Michalsen, MD, professor of integrative medicine at the Institute of Social Medicine, Epidemiology, and Health Economics of the Charité University Medical Center in Berlin and director of the Department of Internal and Integrative Medicine at the Immanuel Hospital in Berlin; Hanno Pijl, MD, internist-endocrinologist in the Department of Internal Medicine of the Leiden University Medical Center in the Netherlands and professor of diabetology at Leiden University; and Mauro Frigeri, MD, oncologist and expert in palliative care at the Ticino Hospice Foundation in Lugano, Switzerland.

BREAST CANCER: WHAT IT IS AND HOW IT IS TREATED

Breast cancer, the cancer most commonly diagnosed in women, has been by far the most studied in combination with fasting and fasting-mimicking diets, in both the laboratory and hospitals around the world (figure 4.1). Thanks to this international effort and to the positive results of recent randomized clinical studies combining fasting-mimicking diets with chemotherapy to treat breast cancer, we are hopefully close to a day when fasting-mimicking diets will be used in combination with a variety of therapies to treat breast cancer.

There are three main types of breast cancers:[1]

Hormone receptor (HR) positive. HR-positive cancer cells have either the estrogen receptor, a protein that is activated by the estrogen hormone, or the progesterone receptor, activated by progesterone, or both. Estrogen is the hormone responsible for the development of female physical features (breasts and female genitals), menstrual cycle, and pregnancy, as well as many other tissue-specific effects in both sexes. In HR-positive breast cancers, these hormone pathways are very active and contribute to the cancer's survival and growth. These cancers are treated with hormone therapy to block the action of hormones.

Human epidermal growth factor receptor 2 (HER2) positive. These cancer cells contain a receptor that is activated in response to the presence of another molecule that promotes growth: the epidermal growth factor. Patients with this type of breast cancer can be (a) hormone receptor positive (HR positive, see above) or (b) HR negative, meaning that no estrogen or progesterone receptor is present. These cancers are treated with drugs that target the growth factor HER2, often in combination with chemotherapy or endocrine therapy (for HR-positive cases).

Triple negative. These cancers, which are among the most aggressive, have neither the estrogen or progesterone hormone receptors nor the HER2 receptor and are mainly cured with surgery and chemotherapy and occasionally with immunotherapy added to chemotherapy.

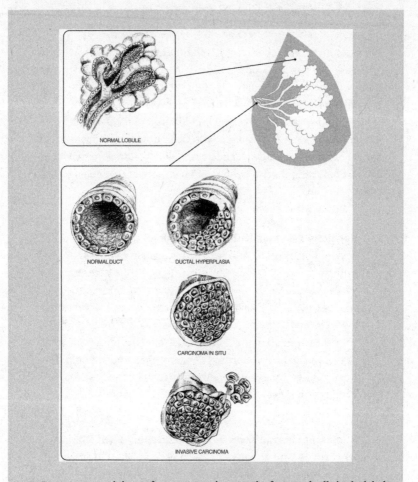

NORMAL LOBULE

NORMAL DUCT

DUCTAL HYPERPLASIA

CARCINOMA IN SITU

INVASIVE CARCINOMA

4.1. *Breast cancer originates from an excessive growth of mutated cells in the lobule (area in the gland that produces milk). When the cancer is in situ, tumoral cells have not invaded the nearby tissues or other body parts. In invasive cancer, cells have grown so much that they have outgrown the lobule.*

I BELIEVE MOST PATIENTS AND their doctors are choosing either the standard drug-based approach (supported by virtually all oncologists) or alternative approaches, including dietary restrictions (generally either opposed or dismissed by oncologists). As someone who collaborates with many leading oncologists around the world, I can tell you that those who eschew alternative approaches are not doing so to protect drug sales. Rather, most of them are not aware of the nutrition literature or trained in nutrition or other integrative approaches. They may also view dietary restriction as ineffective and potentially harmful to patients, and they are very careful before making changes that are not considered "standard of care," which in most cases is based on approval by the FDA. Are they wrong? Technically no, but they may not be doing what could be most effective for patients, especially those in advanced stages of the disease.

Clearly, the standard of care monitored by the regulatory agencies is there to protect patients, and the argument oncologists make is that fasting-mimicking diets need to be tested further before they can be deemed more universally acceptable in clinical practice. Until then, how do doctors and patients who want to use a more integrative approach to nutrition in cancer therapy solve this dilemma? The best strategy is to be respectful of the standard of care and use nutrition as a support and not a replacement, at least until enough clinical data is available to include nutrition in the standard of care. I don't say this as a way to compromise, but in twenty years of research by my lab and many others, we have consistently seen that only the combination of cancer drugs with fasting or fasting-mimicking diets led to cancer-free survival in mice and a potentially higher effectiveness and less toxicity of the therapy in humans. This is particularly clear for breast cancer but also for other cancer types for which we rarely observe that fasting/fasting-mimicking diets cause regression in mice without also using drugs.

Around 2012, I was presenting at a workshop in Germany and one of the leading German oncologists stopped my presentation and told the audience that I had not even begun to demonstrate that fasting and fasting-mimicking diets make cancer therapy more effective. I responded, "If you were bitten by a cobra and I had an antidote that (1) was effective against cobra venom in mice and (2) was shown to be safe, but no one knew if it was effective in humans, would you take it?" He did not respond, but he knew, and we all knew, the answer was yes.

I use this example because a cobra bite is well recognized as lethal, so death would be unavoidable. Although an oncologist, together with a registered dietitian or other nutrition professional, could recommend fasting-mimicking diets for cancer patients at any stage, in advanced-stage cases and when the viable options have limited efficacy, oncologists can be respectful of standard of care while giving the patient an additional chance of survival based on solid science.

NUTRITECHNOLOGY AND ITS ROLE AGAINST BREAST CANCER AND OTHER TUMORS

Nutrition was and still is viewed by many doctors as a "palliative" intervention, not really effective against the disease but possibly helpful to make the patient feel better or more involved in their care. Fasting and the fasting-mimicking diet are viewed the same way and get the same treatment as "fruits and vegetables" or "having a healthy diet." Thus, I started using the terms *nutritechnology*, *differential stress resistance* (DSR) (focused on increasing protection of normal but not cancer cells from therapy), and *differential stress sensitization* (DSS) (focused on increasing the killing of cancer cells by the therapy) to make it clear we were not talking about nutritional changes that are there to nourish or cause only small improvements. Our research supports a very specific type of fasting-mimicking and nutrition plan in which the number of calories, each ingredient, and the frequency of the diet cycles must be carefully designed to achieve strong anticancer effects, especially in combination with cancer drugs.

Nutritechnology has nothing to do with a "healthy diet" but has much to do with the many molecular changes that are often very different or even opposite between normal and cancer cells and that can match and even surpass the potency of cancer drugs, at least in mice. One major reason for this is the ability of the fasting-mimicking diet to trigger many coordinated changes, which lead to the death of cancer cells while often protecting normal cells from toxic drugs. These wide changes are extremely important for breast cancer cells for two major reasons: First, as normal cells transform into breast cancer cells, their energy requirements increase, and they become dependent on a combination of nutrients and growth factors, with different types of breast cancer cells requiring different combinations of these. Second, in most cases, eventually the breast cancer cells become resistant to the drugs used against them.

For example, a breast cancer mass may be initially sensitive to the drug doxorubicin, widely used in therapy to target breast cancer cells. Eventually, some cells within that mass (that were either already present within the cancer or are newly formed) become resistant not only to doxorubicin but also to the moderate changes in glucose levels that can be achieved in the patient. This situation can be problematic, because by this point the patient has received many cycles of chemotherapy, which has killed cancer cells but also damaged normal cells and organs and made the patient frail. Second, the cancer is no longer responding to either the drug or the limited (low-glucose) diet. In fact, in a recent paper in the journal *Nature,* the authors pointed out how cancer cells change and evolve during therapy and how within a few months the cancer can be different from the original one.[2] To give you an analogy, imagine a grassy area with weeds feeding on water and nutrients that also feed the grass. A weed killer is used, but it also damages the grass, although not as severely as the weeds. At first the attempt is successful: the weeds disappear, and the grass survives. However, eventually the grass will become sick and die from the pesticide, while the weeds will become resistant and take over the field. The weeds, like the cancer cells becoming resistant to the therapy, eventually generate a variant that no longer dies when exposed to the weed killer. To explain how this works, in the next section I will describe our experiments in mice as well as our clinical results.

Fasting and Fasting-Mimicking Diets in Breast Cancer and Chemotherapy Treatment

In 2008, we published our findings on fasting's ability to shield mice's healthy cells but not cancer cells. After the publication, oncologists asked, "Interesting, but are you sure you are not also protecting cancer cells?" We told them that we expected that the fasting would not only not protect cancer cells but might also make them more sensitive to chemotherapy. And three years later, we proved it: With the help of graduate student Changhan Lee in my lab in Los Angeles and researcher Lizzia Raffaghello at the Gaslini children's hospital in Italy, we showed that fasting

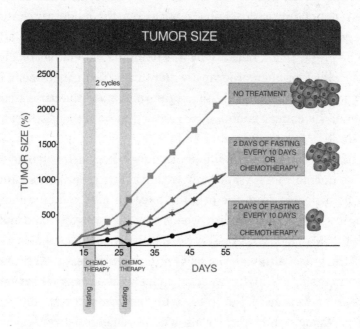

4.2. *Tumor progression in mice with breast cancer. Two fasting cycles alone are as effective as two chemotherapy cycles. However, two cycles of fasting combined with chemotherapy are much more effective than chemo alone, even fifty-five days after the start. Modified from Changhan Lee et al., "Fasting Cycles Retard Growth of Tumors and Sensitize a Range of Cancer Cell Types to Chemotherapy,"* Science Translational Medicine 4, no. 124 (2012): 124ra27.

made a variety of cancer cells, including both human and mouse breast cancer cells, much more sensitive to chemotherapy. Notably, cycles of fasting alone were as effective against breast cancer as cycles of chemotherapy, as shown in the graph (figure 4.2).

In another type of breast cancer, whose cells were obtained many years ago from a patient and grown in the laboratory (MDA-MB-231), results were very different between fasting alone and fasting plus chemotherapy.

We observed the following:

1. Tumor measurements from mice that were fed normally (control group) and treated with the chemotherapy drug were terminated at day 11, because all of the mice had died from chemotherapy (DXR or doxorubicin, a chemotherapeutic drug) toxicity (figure 4.3).

2. The growth of the breast tumor was delayed during fasting, but after refeeding, the tumor appeared to grow even faster than under the standard diet. This accelerated post-fasting cancer growth may be the result of overfeeding, weight gain, and high growth factor levels in mice that were allowed to eat without restrictions between fasting cycles.

3. However, when fasting was combined with chemotherapy, the progression of the human breast cancer tumors was dramatically delayed, and the tumor did not progress (figure 4.3). When we started with a relatively low number of the very aggressive triple-negative breast cancer cells, none of the mice receiving either chemotherapy or fasting cycles alone were cured, but up to 60 percent of the mice receiving both chemotherapy and fasting cycles remained without cancer for very long periods of time and were likely free of cancer.

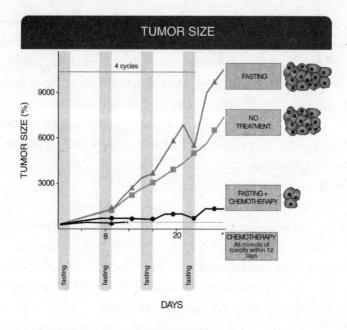

4.3. *Chemotherapy reduces cancer growth but becomes toxic after a certain period of time, leading to mouse death. Cancer grows rapidly when (1) no treatment is used or (2) only fasting is administered. But when fasting is combined with chemotherapy, cancer progression is drastically slowed down, and this together with the reduced toxicity to the mouse results in long-term survival. Modified from Changhan Lee et al.,* "Fasting Cycles Retard Growth of Tumors and Sensitize a Range of Cancer Cell Types to Chemotherapy," *Science Translational Medicine 4, no. 124 (2012): 124ra27.*

Fasting and Fasting-Mimicking Diets Cause Immunotherapy-Like Effects

Immunotherapy, which entails the use of drugs called immune checkpoint inhibitors to promote the attack of cancer cells by cells of the immune system, is among the most effective therapies against some tumors. One of the most promising areas of cancer research, immunotherapy resulted in the Nobel Prize in Physiology or Medicine being awarded to James P. Allison and Tasuku Honjo, who first described it in experimental models.

Could fasting or the fasting-mimicking diet generate its own "immunotherapy" effect and thereby turn the immune system against cancer cells? When Stefano Di Biase analyzed triple-negative breast tumor masses in my laboratory at USC in Los Angeles, he saw that in the mice that had undergone fasting-mimicking-diet cycles in combination with chemotherapy, immune cells had penetrated the tumor masses and were killing the cancer cells (figure 4.4). However, this did not happen in mice that received chemotherapy while on a standard diet or on the fasting-mimicking diet alone. Thus, the fasting-mimicking diet helped activate immune cells, which then attacked and helped neutralize cancer cells. This is particularly important as fasting-mimicking diets are nontoxic and can be tolerated for many cycles, unlike chemotherapy or immunotherapy, which cause severe side effects.

It is worth stressing that as of now, immunotherapy alone seems to have a limited effectiveness on breast cancer. But fasting-mimicking-diet studies show that it makes immunotherapy much more effective against breast cancer in mice.

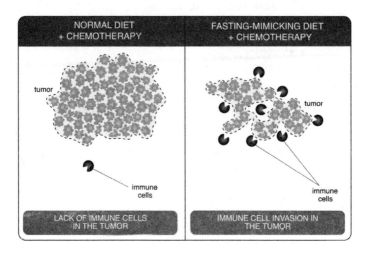

4.4. *The reorganization of the tumor and immune system during regular nutrition (left) and a fasting-mimicking diet plus chemotherapy (right). The combination of the fasting-mimicking diet with chemotherapy but not each alone increases the level of immune system cells, which recognize and kill cancer cells, thus delaying cancer progression. Modified from Stefano Di Biase et al., "Fasting-Mimicking Diet Reduces HO-1 to Promote T Cell–Mediated Tumor Cytotoxicity,"* Cancer Cell *30, no. 1 (July 11, 2016): 136–46.*

Because cancer immunotherapy is extremely expensive and often accompanied by major side effects, it is important to determine whether fasting-mimicking diets can improve the effect of immunotherapy, reduce its side effects, and perhaps even replace it, at least for the treatment of certain cancers, thus potentially providing an inexpensive alternative to this powerful intervention.

More recently, my laboratory has shown similar results when combining immunotherapy with a fasting-mimicking diet against the very aggressive triple-negative breast cancer in mice. The combination of two immunotherapy drugs with fasting-mimicking-diet cycles was much more effective than the immunotherapy alone against this type of breast cancer, which is known to not be responsive to immunotherapy.[3]

Clinical Trials on Fasting-Mimicking Diets, Nutrition, and Breast Cancer

Although laboratory studies provide the foundation for new cancer therapies, only clinical trials can prove that a new therapy is effective but also test its safety and feasibility. Because the media focuses on positive studies, most people do not realize that the great majority of clinical trials testing new drugs fail because the drugs are found to be ineffective or toxic. Very few make it to FDA approval. Thus, there is great potential in combining fasting-mimicking diets with a wide variety of cancer drugs to make them more effective and/or less toxic against many cancer types and patients.

TRIAL NUMBER 1. HER2-NEGATIVE, STAGE II/III BREAST CANCER

The first clinical trial in which fasting was combined with chemotherapy in breast cancer patients was a small one with thirteen HER2-negative, stage II/III patients, performed at the Leiden University Medical Center, in the Netherlands.[4] HER2-negative cancer cells have low levels or the absence of a growth-factor protein called HER2. This protein helps control cell growth in normal cells. HER2-negative cancer cells may grow more slowly and are less likely to recur or spread to other parts of the body than HER-positive cancer cells. Stage II means that the cancer is present in the breast or in the nearby lymph nodes or in both. Stage III describes a cancer that has spread from the breast to lymph nodes close to it or to the skin of the breast or to the chest wall, but not to distant organs.

The study showed that normal blood cells in patients who fasted prior to treatment were protected from chemotherapy toxicity, and their DNA damage was reduced or reversed. These results provided initial evidence that fasting and fasting-mimicking diets could protect patients from chemotherapy side effects (figure 4.5).

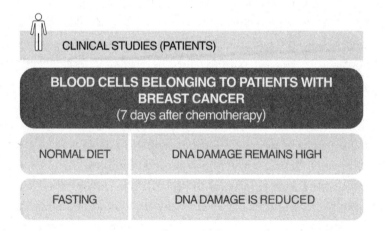

4.5. *Blood cells in patients with breast cancer who have fasted for two days (1) were protected from the toxicity of chemotherapy and (2) were protected from DNA damage, suggesting that fasting and fasting-mimicking diets can protect against some side effects of chemotherapy. Modified from Stefanie de Groot et al., "The Effects of Short-Term Fasting on Tolerance to (Neo) Adjuvant Chemotherapy in HER2-Negative Breast Cancer Patients: A Randomized Pilot Study,"* BMC Cancer *15 (2015): 625.*

TRIAL NUMBER 2. BREAST/OVARIAN CANCER

In another clinical trial, performed by Dr. Michalsen and colleagues at the Charité University Hospital in Berlin, Germany, thirty-four women with breast or ovarian cancer received a modified and very low calorie fasting-mimicking diet for 2.5 days in combination with chemotherapy (thirty-six hours before and twenty-four hours after). The study showed an improvement in various measurements of quality of life and reduction in fatigue.[5] This trial was consistent with trial number 1 and confirmed that fasting can reduce chemotherapy side effects and improve patients' quality of life.

TRIAL NUMBER 3. HER2-NEGATIVE STAGE II/III BREAST CANCER

The initial set of trials, including our own at USC in Los Angeles, had focused on the effect of water-only fasting on cancer therapy. However, given health concerns associated with water-only fasting, including the risk of low blood sugar, blood pressure, sodium levels, etc., it's normally not allowed outside of specialized clinics where patients can be closely monitored. In addition to the safety concerns, this stringent diet is difficult to follow and consequently it was hard to recruit patients for the trials—it took years. But thanks in part to grants by the National Cancer Institute and the National Institute on Aging of the U.S. National Institutes of Health during 2010–2015, we developed the fasting-mimicking diet for the purpose of matching—and possibly surpassing—the effects of water-only fasting while allowing patients to eat regular meals (but with far fewer calories than usual). The development of the fasting-mimicking diet paved the way for the standardization of the fasting method, and the clinics that tested it could give patients the same fasting-mimicking diet, helping guarantee its efficacy.

One of the most important cancer clinical trials on the fasting-mimicking diet was carried out at the Leiden University Medical Center in the Netherlands. It was the largest trial focused on the fasting-mimicking diet and breast cancer, with 131 patients with HER2-negative stage II/III breast cancer, without diabetes and with a BMI over 18 (underweight women were excluded), receiving either the fasting-mimicking diet or their regular diet for three days prior to and one day after chemotherapy. Six to eight chemotherapy cycles were given to them prior to surgery to remove the tumor. For this trial, the oncologists decided to omit glucocorticoid dexamethasone—a steroid used to prevent allergic reactions and nausea from chemotherapy—in the fasting-mimicking diet group, since we had seen that dexamethasone increased glucose (sugar) levels, leading to higher sensitivity and death in the mice receiving chemotherapy.[6] Despite the absence of dexamethasone, side effects did not increase in patients receiving the fasting-mimicking diet, providing initial evidence that the fasting-mimicking diet can safely replace dexamethasone in reducing certain side effects. In addition, the DNA damage caused by chemotherapy was reduced in the immune cells of those doing the fasting-mimicking diet, as shown in the previous water-only-fasting trial (trial number 1).

More important, patients receiving the fasting-mimicking diet in combination with chemotherapy showed remarkable effects on their cancer cells. The portion of patients for whom the chemotherapy was not effective (no tumor shrinkage) was nearly three times smaller among those who completed any cycles of the fasting-mimicking diet and over five times smaller in patients who combined the fasting-mimicking diet with chemotherapy for at least half of the cycles (fasting-mimicking diet compliant, those who were able to complete the FMD in at least half of the chemo cycles) (figure 4.6). This response was determined by radiology: magnetic resonance imaging (MRI) and ultrasound.

These radiology results (CT scan, etc.) matched the pathology results obtained by analyzing the tumor cells removed during surgery. In fact, 45 percent of the masses removed from patients who combined most chemo cycles with the fasting-mimicking diet were 90 to 100 percent cancer free, whereas only 20 percent of the masses removed from patients receiving chemotherapy while on a regular diet were 90 to 100 percent cancer free (figure 4.7).

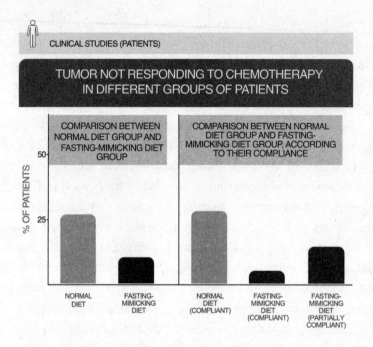

CLINICAL STUDIES (PATIENTS)

TUMOR NOT RESPONDING TO CHEMOTHERAPY IN DIFFERENT GROUPS OF PATIENTS

COMPARISON BETWEEN NORMAL DIET GROUP AND FASTING-MIMICKING DIET GROUP

COMPARISON BETWEEN NORMAL DIET GROUP AND FASTING-MIMICKING DIET GROUP, ACCORDING TO THEIR COMPLIANCE

% OF PATIENTS

50

25

NORMAL DIET

FASTING-MIMICKING DIET

NORMAL DIET (COMPLIANT)

FASTING-MIMICKING DIET (COMPLIANT)

FASTING-MIMICKING DIET (PARTIALLY COMPLIANT)

4.6. *The percentage of patients for whom chemotherapy was ineffective was five times lower in patients receiving chemotherapy and completing at least half of those cycles with the fasting-mimicking diet versus those receiving the chemotherapy with a normal diet. Modified from Stefanie de Groot et al., "Fasting-Mimicking Diet as an Adjunct to Neoadjuvant Chemotherapy for Breast Cancer in the Multicentre Randomized Phase 2 DIRECT Trial,"* Nature Communications *11, no. 1 (June 23, 2020): 3083.*

Remarkably, the more fasting-mimicking-diet cycles were done, the better the response in the patients (figure 4.8).

This trial also demonstrated how well the fasting-mimicking diet causes changes in patients, such as an increase in ketone bodies, i.e., ketogenesis (ketone bodies are water-soluble molecules *produced by the liver in response to fasting*), as well as the lowering of glucose, insulin, and IGF-1, changes known to reduce cancer survival and growth—as we have later confirmed in two additional clinical trials (see the following section and figure 4.9).[7] In summary, the first relatively large, randomized study on the use of the fasting-mimicking diet and cancer progression, which included 131 patients, is very promising, especially considering the effects

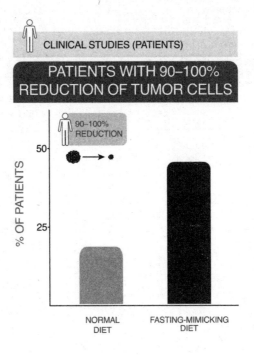

4.7. *Masses that were removed from patients who underwent chemotherapy were 90 to 100 percent free of cancer cells (1) in 45 percent of patients who were administered chemotherapy and the fasting-mimicking diet and (2) in 20 percent of patients who underwent chemotherapy following a regular diet. Modified from Stefanie de Groot et al., "Fasting-Mimicking Diet as an Adjunct to Neoadjuvant Chemotherapy for Breast Cancer in the Multicentre Randomized Phase 2 DIRECT Trial,"* Nature Communications *11, no. 1 (June 23, 2020): 3083.*

of the fasting-mimicking diet and chemotherapy on tumor mass size and the survival of active cancer cells. Notably, whereas over 80 percent of patients completed at least one cycle of the fasting-mimicking diet, fewer than 50 percent completed three or more cycles of the fasting-mimicking diet. I believe this was mostly because (1) the nutritionists in the many Dutch centers conducting the test were not familiar with fasting and the fasting-mimicking diet and may not have been familiar with dietary restrictions (training in the cancer nutrition community recommends that patients eat more, not less) and (2) patients may have associated a particular food in the fasting-mimicking diet with the side effects of

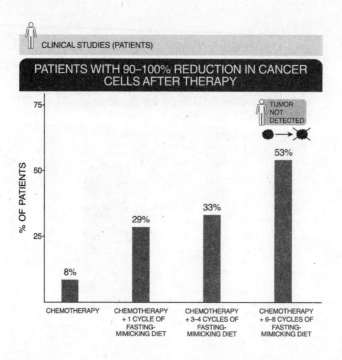

CLINICAL STUDIES (PATIENTS)

4.8. *The 90 to 100 percent tumor free masses have been observed (1) only in 8 percent of patients who completed chemotherapy without any cycle of the fasting-mimicking diet; (2) in 29 percent of those who completed chemotherapy with only one cycle of the fasting-mimicking diet; (3) in 33 percent of those who completed chemotherapy with three or four cycles of the fasting-mimicking diet; and (4) in 53 percent of those who combined all chemotherapy cycles with the fasting-mimicking diet. Modified from Stefanie de Groot et al., "Fasting-Mimicking Diet as an Adjunct to Neoadjuvant Chemotherapy for Breast Cancer in the Multicentre Randomized Phase 2 DIRECT Trial,"* Nature Communications 11, no. 1 *(June 23, 2020): 3083.*

chemotherapy, thus finding it difficult to continue to consume that particular food (food aversion). This points to the need to develop a wider variety of foods in the fasting-mimicking diet.

TRIAL NUMBERS 4 AND 5. HORMONE
THERAPIES AND BREAST CANCER

Approximately 75 percent of all breast cancer cells grow and survive in part thanks to the proliferative (growth-stimulating) effects of hormones, primarily estrogen. Thus, antihormonal therapy, in which drugs are used to block the effects of these hormones,

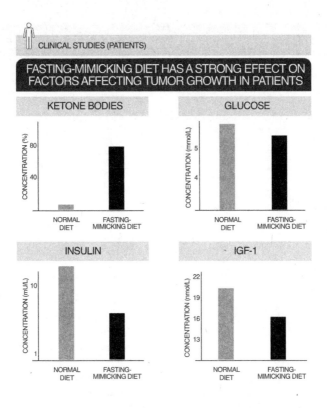

4.9. *During the fasting-mimicking diet, ketone bodies (generated from fat to be used as fuel) increase, while glucose, insulin, and IGF-1 levels decrease and are lower than their levels on a normal diet. These changes can reduce cancer growth and cancer-cell survival. Modified from Stefanie de Groot et al., "Fasting-Mimicking Diet as an Adjunct to Neoadjuvant Chemotherapy for Breast Cancer in the Multicentre Randomized Phase 2 DIRECT Trial,"* Nature Communications *11, no. 1 (June 23, 2020): 3083.*

is often used to halt cancer progression. Unfortunately, these cancers can become resistant to such hormone-blocking therapy and resume growth. Recently, in collaboration with Professor Nencioni's laboratory at the University of Genoa in Italy, my laboratory at IFOM in Milan showed that hormone therapy, plus an additional biologically targeted drug called palbociclib, could prevent hormone-dependent breast cancer growth for several months in mice, but eventually, as in patients, cancer cells became resistant to this therapy and grew. Also, the anticancer hormone therapy induced abnormal endometrial growth (the endometrium is the

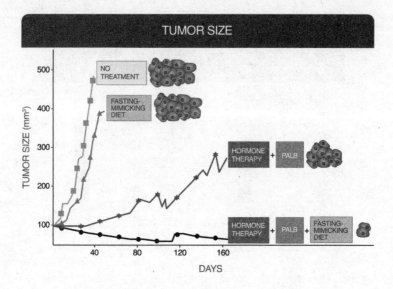

4.10. A. *Hormonal therapy with palbociclib (a targeted drug for the treatment of breast cancer that is HR positive and HER2 negative) blocks breast cancer growth for several months in mice, but in the long term, cancer cells become resistant to this therapy and grow. When the fasting-mimicking diet is added to this treatment, the combination stops cancer from becoming resistant to drugs and, consequently, causes the cancer to regress and many mice to become cancer free. Modified from Irene Caffa et al., "Fasting-Mimicking Diet and Hormone Therapy Induce Breast Cancer Regression," Nature 583, no. 7817 (2020): 620–24.*

mucous membrane lining the uterus) in women treated with this class of hormone therapy. Fasting and fasting-mimicking-diet cycles not only prevented cancer from becoming resistant to the hormone-therapy drugs and prevented the abnormal endometrial growth but also were able to reverse cancer growth after cancer cells had become resistant to the drugs in mice (figure 4.10, A and B).

The same publication also included thirty-six breast cancer patients receiving hormone therapy from two different clinical trials: one carried out at the San Martino Hospital in Genoa and the other at the Italian National Cancer Institute in Milan.[8] Although these are not randomized clinical trials, the results from these patients are providing very promising data in support of the safety

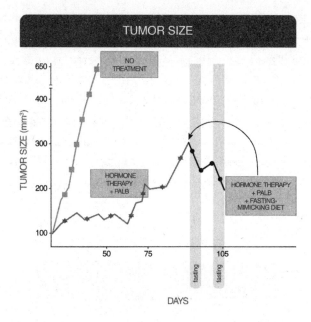

4.10. B. *Fasting-mimicking-diet cycles were able to cause a reduction in tumor size in mice after cancer cells became resistant to drugs. Modified from Irene Caffa et al., "Fasting-Mimicking Diet and Hormone Therapy Induce Breast Cancer Regression,"* Nature 583, no. 7817 (2020): 620–24.

and potential effectiveness of the fasting-mimicking diet in combination with hormone therapy, which will need to be confirmed in randomized trials.

As observed in mice, fasting-mimicking-diet cycles caused the reduction of the following factors: insulin, leptin, and IGF-1 (which promotes cell—even cancer cell—proliferation). This outcome has a very high clinical significance because these three factors were responsible for the resistance to hormone therapy and growth of breast cancer cells demonstrated in the mouse studies, so their reduction is expected to negatively affect cancer survival and growth in humans.

In the trial at San Martino Hospital in Genoa, patients received a five-day fasting-mimicking diet every four weeks. They completed an average of seven fasting-mimicking-diet cycles, with some undergoing up to fourteen cycles. As in the previous trials listed above, the fasting-mimicking diet proved to be safe, leading to only minor side effects including headache (41 percent) and fatigue (21 percent). Patients from the study in Milan received a similar five-day fasting-mimicking diet every three to four weeks and completed an average of five and a half cycles with no severe adverse events.

Patients from the trial in Genoa, who also received dietary recommendations and instructions for daily muscle training for the intervals between fasting-mimicking-diet cycles (figure 4.11),

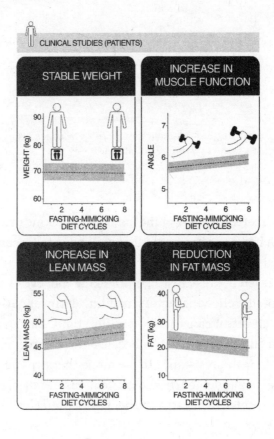

4.11. *Patients who received and followed dietary and muscle-training recommendations in between the fasting-mimicking diets kept their body weight stable, increased markers consistent with higher muscle function, increased their muscle mass, and decreased their fat mass over time. Modified from Irene Caffa et al., "Fasting-Mimicking Diet and Hormone Therapy Induce Breast Cancer Regression,"* Nature *583, no. 7817 (2020).*

maintained a stable body weight and handgrip strength but also showed increases in muscle function and muscle mass over time, whereas their fat mass decreased. Notably, patients received recommendations to follow a relatively high-protein and high-starch Mediterranean diet between fasting-mimicking-diet cycles, which, in combination with weight training, would explain the increase in muscle function and mass.

However, since the purpose of these therapies was not to cause an increase in muscle function and mass but rather to maintain them while attacking the cancer, patients should work closely with a nutritionist or physician and follow the everyday dietary and muscle-exercise recommendations described in chapter 3 while monitoring (1) muscle function (tested by measurement of phase angle), (2) muscle mass (tested by DEXA scan), (3) grip strength, (4) weight / body mass index (BMI), and (5) abdominal circumference. The medical team should ensure that patients consume a diet that keeps low the levels of certain blood amino acids (through low to moderate plant-based proteins) and sugars (through low dietary starches and sugars), without compromising patients' ability to maintain a normal weight and muscle/bone mass. This is not easy to achieve, but it is done routinely at the Create Cures Foundation clinic and can be achieved by other qualified health-care teams.

As discussed, (1) high intake of protein / amino acids increases IGF-1 and insulin levels, and (2) refined carbohydrates and sugars increase the levels of blood glucose and insulin. IGF-1, insulin, and glucose can help a wide range of tumors survive and grow (figure 4.12).

TRIAL NUMBER 6. TRIPLE-NEGATIVE
BREAST CANCER: LONG-TERM SURVIVAL

Ultimately, any new therapy that is truly effective must extend the average survival of the patients receiving that new therapy compared with the previous standard therapy. This is particularly important for one of the most common and aggressive cancers: triple-negative breast cancer. Dr. Claudio Vernieri, of the National

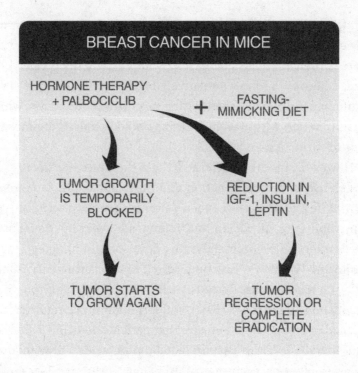

BREAST CANCER IN MICE

HORMONE THERAPY
+ PALBOCICLIB

+ FASTING-
MIMICKING DIET

TUMOR GROWTH
IS TEMPORARILY
BLOCKED

REDUCTION IN
IGF-1, INSULIN,
LEPTIN

TUMOR STARTS
TO GROW AGAIN

TUMOR
REGRESSION OR
COMPLETE
ERADICATION

4.12. *In mice, the fasting-mimicking diet lowers insulin, IGF-1, and leptin levels, which makes hormone therapy and chemotherapy more effective against cancer growth (right). Modified from Irene Caffa et al., "Fasting-Mimicking Diet and Hormone Therapy Induce Breast Cancer Regression,"* Nature *583, no. 7817 (2020): 620–24.*

Tumor Institute in Milan, and his colleagues compared the overall survival of fourteen advanced-stage triple-negative breast cancer patients receiving chemotherapy (carboplatin-gemcitabine) plus cycles of the fasting-mimicking diet with the overall survival of seventy-six triple-negative breast cancer patients treated with the same chemotherapy alone at the Italian National Cancer Institute. Patients undergoing cycles of a fasting-mimicking diet in combination with chemotherapy on average survived nearly twice as long as patients receiving chemotherapy alone (average survival was 30.3 months for patients receiving the fasting-mimicking diet plus chemotherapy versus 17.2 months for those receiving

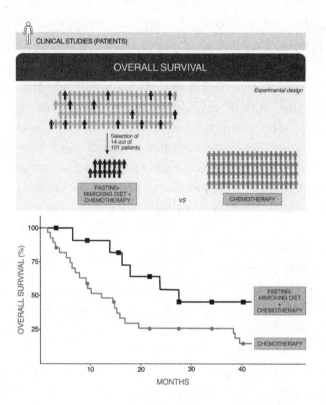

4.13. *Median long-term survival in months is more than doubled in breast cancer patients receiving fasting-mimicking-diet cycles plus chemotherapy compared with those receiving chemotherapy alone.*

chemotherapy alone) (figure 4.13). At 40 months the portion of patients surviving was over twice as high in the group receiving fasting-mimicking diet cycles plus chemotherapy versus those receiving chemotherapy alone (35.7 percent versus 15.7 percent).[9]

ADDITIONAL CLINICAL TRIALS

Stefanie Zorn and colleagues have also performed a clinical trial on fasting and breast and ovarian cancers that shows promising results. (I discuss the trial in the following chapter on gynecological cancers.)[10]

Another study on the benefit of fasting in cancer patients

evaluated restrictive diets and fasting practices in about 2,700 cancer survivors. The analysis of questionnaires completed by the patients revealed that after cancer diagnosis, 3.5 percent of patients added some form of fasting to their standard therapies. Patients reported that in their opinion fasting strongly improved cancer prognosis.[11] The motivation among breast cancer patients to fast is mainly the desire to lower the negative side effects of chemotherapy. Interestingly, fasting seems to reduce anxiety among patients, since it is associated with a greater sense of control over their treatment. This study also raises the possibility that patients not supported by their doctors on this nutritional strategy may turn to complementary health-care practitioners.[12]

The data gathered in the study underscore how important it is to empower the patient as well as prompt their oncologist to form a team able to handle the integration of standard of care with novel and safe complementary therapies that have the potential to render standard treatment more effective.

Both trial numbers 4 and 5 described earlier focused on multiple types of cancers and therapies and had two hundred patients enrolled at either the Italian National Cancer Institute in Milan or the University of Genoa. They confirmed the safety of fasting-mimicking-diet cycles in the treatment of many cancer types and in combination with a range of therapies.[13] Trial number 4 also provided two major findings: (1) It confirmed that fasting-mimicking-diet cycles can increase antitumor activity and increase the infiltration of immune cells in cancer masses. (2) It showed that five advanced-stage patients with lung, colon, breast, and pancreatic cancers (who combined the fasting-mimicking diet with various therapies) went into an unexpected long-term remission, which the oncologists defined as "exceptional responses."[14] Finally, trial number 6 indicates that advanced-stage triple-negative breast cancer patients may live nearly twice as long when chemotherapy is combined with fasting-mimicking-diet cycles, although larger trials are needed to confirm these results (figure 4.13).

. . . .

HERE ARE TWO TRIPLE-NEGATIVE BREAST cancer cases from the five patients showing "exceptional responses" from the study described above:

- The first case is of a fifty-eight-year-old woman diagnosed with stage II triple-negative breast cancer. She received a complex therapy that included a breast-conserving surgery. The surgery was preceded by a therapy (neoadjuvant) and followed by radiation and after-surgery (adjuvant) chemotherapy. Despite this aggressive therapy, a bone scan performed six months after surgery revealed the presence of a metastatic iliac lesion (figure 4.14). After enrolling in the clinical trial coordinated by Dr. Vernieri, she received chemotherapy in combination with eight triweekly cycles of a fasting-mimicking diet, followed by maintenance chemotherapy. Imaging to monitor the tumor size (computed tomography and bone scans) performed at the end of combination therapy revealed complete regression, even thirty-six months after the start of treatment. Moreover, a fasting-mimicking diet led to a significant reduction in serum IGF-1 concentration. Weight loss that occurred during the fasting-mimicking diet was mostly recovered during refeeding periods.

- The second case is of a forty-two-year-old woman with genetic triple-negative breast cancer, since she bears the BRCA1 mutation, with two liver metastases. The patient was enrolled in the same trial and started chemotherapy in combination with fasting-mimicking-diet cycles. She discontinued the fasting-mimicking diet after five cycles due to fatigue and received additional rounds of chemotherapy. Computed tomography and breast magnetic

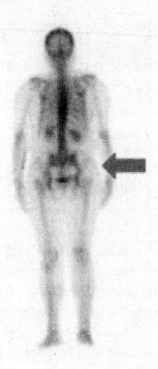

4.14. *Representation of a bone scan performed six months after surgery on a fifty-eight-year-old woman affected by advanced triple-negative breast cancer, which revealed the presence of a metastasis, as indicated by the arrow. After enrollment in the clinical trial, she received chemotherapy in combination with eight triweekly fasting-mimicking-diet cycles, followed by maintenance chemotherapy. The bone scan and the computer tomography scan (not shown) performed at the end of combination therapy revealed radiologic and metabolic complete remission, even thirty-six months after treatment initiation. From Francesca Ligorio et al., "Exceptional Tumour Responses to Fasting-Mimicking Diet Combined with Standard Anticancer Therapies: A Sub-Analysis of the NCT03340935 Trial,"* European Journal of Cancer *172 (September 2022): 300–310.*

resonance imaging (MRI) scans performed after three cycles of treatment revealed an excellent radiological response, and subsequent evaluations performed after ten and seventeen cycles showed a complete response (no evidence of the disease) of both breast and liver lesions (figure 4.15). After around one year, due to repeated episodes of toxicity, the chemotherapy was discontinued. The patient is currently off therapy, with the absence of disease.

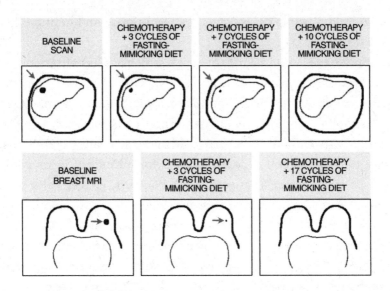

4.15. *Representation of computer tomography (upper panels) and bilateral contrast-enhanced breast MRI (lower panels) scan images at baseline and after three treatment cycles revealed an excellent radiological response in a forty-two-year-old woman with advanced triple-negative breast cancer with BRCA1 mutation. The arrows indicate the liver lesions (upper panels) and the left breast nodule (lower panels). Modified from Francesca Ligorio et al., "Exceptional Tumour Responses to Fasting-Mimicking Diet Combined with Standard Anticancer Therapies: A Sub-Analysis of the NCT03340935 Trial,"* European Journal of Cancer *172 (2022): 300–310.*

FASTING AND STARVATION ESCAPE ROUTES: THE WILD-CARD EFFECT

If you think about cancer research, and how each treatment has a different cellular target, the wide and consistent effects of fasting and the fasting-mimicking diet are very surprising. Immunotherapy is effective only against certain tumors and only in a percentage of patients with that type of tumor. Hormone therapy also works against very specific types of cancer cells, which eventually become resistant to it. What is it about the fasting and the fasting-mimicking diet that gives them the "wild card" effect—making so many cancer therapies (ranging from chemotherapy to kinase inhibitors, radiation, immunotherapy, and hormone therapy) work better (and in some cases, much better) in mice and in initial human trials?

Unlike the great majority of drugs, which are by definition specific and thus expected to work on a specific tumor at a specific stage, fasting and fasting-mimicking diets take advantage of fundamental properties of both normal cells and cancer cells. Normal cells know exactly what to do under starvation conditions, since they have been exposed to them for billions of years going back to their bacterial ancestors. In contrast, cancer cells have evolved in the presence of excess nutrients and under fasting conditions are forced to desperately look for escape routes to survive, since they have acquired so many mutations and DNA changes that they are no longer able to properly handle starvation. They may require more sugar, or more insulin or IGF-1, more ferritin, or more leptin, etc. Notably, every cancer is different. Some may be dependent on high levels of glucose, while others are unaffected by them, and some are very sensitive to insulin levels. But it gets even more complex, as a tumor can initially be sensitive to low glucose levels but then lose this weakness by acquiring mutations or other DNA changes and subsequently become resistant to low glucose and sensitive to low insulin or low IGF-1. In our hormone therapy and breast cancer study we observed that only one of the three different factors lowered by the fasting-mimicking diet (insulin, leptin, and IGF-1) was sufficient for cancer cells to survive and grow.

In our 2021 study[15] led by Giulia Salvadori in my laboratory at IFOM in Milan, we realized that this desperate attempt by cancer cells to find ways to survive in response to the fasting-mimicking diet could be exploited (1) to move away from toxic drugs like chemotherapy, and even immunotherapy, and (2) to use less toxic or nontoxic inhibitors that block specific metabolic pathways activated by cancer cells in an attempt to survive fasting and fasting-mimicking diet conditions (we call these "starvation escape pathways," or SEPs).

When we examine cancer cells at the molecular level, we can't see which sets of genes (pathways) are the most important for survival. However, when we apply the fasting-mimicking diet, cancer cells desperately activate a limited number of starvation escape pathways key for survival. In our 2020 study[16] on hormone therapy and cancer, we focused on human cancer cells and showed how using specific drugs to target the pathways that remain active after treatment with fasting and the fasting-mimicking diet is sufficient not only to prevent cancer growth but also to rapidly reverse growing tumors. In other words, the fasting-mimicking diet reduces the escape pathways, and the remaining ones can be easily hit with appropriate drugs.

Imagine if the police wanted to catch thieves who have been robbing grocery stores in a farming town (figure 4.16). Since the police don't know the identities of the thieves, they make a plan to catch them by closing all the grocery stores. Most of the people in the town can live off their own field's crops, but the thieves do not know how to farm and don't have food reserves, so they are forced to leave to find an open grocery store in a neighboring town. The police put roadblocks in place, confront anyone attempting to leave town, and ultimately identify and stop the thieves. Cancer cells are the thieves, unable to store or grow the food; normal cells are the farmers who can survive without outside food sources; the closing of the grocery stores by the police represents the starvation period imposed by the fasting-mimicking diet; the roads used by thieves to look for food represent the escape routes that cancer cells take to obtain food needed to survive under starvation conditions; and the police roadblocks represent the drugs used to block the starvation escape routes. We can treat cancer in very much the same way these cops catch robbers.

Although we have used this system only for several types of cancer in mice, the use of the fasting-mimicking diet has the potential to be applicable to many cancers against which drugs alone are not sufficient. So Giulia Salvadori and the rest of my team

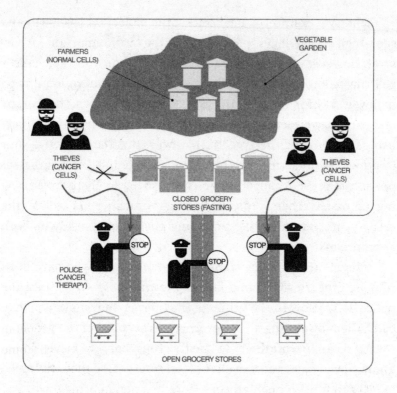

4.16. *This example compares food-stealing thieves to cancer. The "starving" of cancer cells can be imagined as the closure of grocery stores in town. With these conditions, farmers (normal cells) can survive without buying food, thanks to the food grown on their land (autophagy process). Thieves (cancer cells) cannot store food and try to take the escape routes to reach other towns and find food to survive, but they are stopped by the police (therapy with different drugs).*

were able to identify the escape pathways and use relatively low-toxicity drugs to cause long-term tumor regression in mice with triple-negative breast cancer, raising the possibility that soon we will be able to use this system to identify standard and already FDA-approved drugs (approved for other uses) that when combined with the fasting-mimicking diet can cause the same effect in humans.

• • • • • •

A WORD OF CAUTION FOR
CANCER PATIENTS

Like all other cancer therapies, including chemotherapy and immunotherapy, the emerging fasting-mimicking-diet cycles are not a magical intervention that will cure or improve therapy against all cancers at all stages. Thus, cancer patients for whom standard therapy is expected to bring high survival/cure rates may consider adopting the Longevity Diet and other lifestyle changes but not the periodic fasting-mimicking-diet cycles.

Each patient should talk to their oncologist and consider the fasting-mimicking diet at all stages. We don't have any evidence that the fasting-mimicking diet causes the standard cancer drugs to be less effective, but it is possible. A patient who has a 95 percent chance of being cured by surgery combined with chemo may be taking an unnecessary risk by adding the fasting-mimicking diet to the therapy, at least until more clinical data become available.

It would be a very different scenario for an advanced-stage metastatic cancer patient whose survival chances are slim because there are no effective therapies currently available. This was the situation of the patients showing "exceptional responses" in the advanced-stage cancers in the Ligorio study described above.[17] It was also true for the advanced-stage triple-negative breast cancer patients described earlier, among whom the percentage of patients who received the fasting-mimicking-diet cycles alive after forty months of treatment was more than doubled compared to those who received chemo alone (figure 4.13). With such advanced-stage cancers, patients should definitely discuss with their oncologist adding the fasting-mimicking diet to the standard-of-care therapy.

. . . .

THE LONGEVITY DIET DURING
BREAST CANCER THERAPY

In our 2021 study in mice, we confirmed that the level of sugar in the blood affects the progression of metastatic breast cancer. These results are consistent with those of 1,261 patients with non-metastatic breast cancer studied in 2019 by the Italian National Cancer Institute in Milan, indicating that patients with glucose levels below 87 mg/dl are approximately half as likely to have distant metastases as those with higher glucose levels.[18] The risk of recurrence and death was also higher in patients with higher glucose levels, especially when considering only overweight women. The medical team, including the oncologist, should help patients maintain low levels of glucose, protein, and consequently amino acids, without causing malnourishment and loss of muscle and bone mass. Not surprisingly, in a study of 2,413 breast cancer patients, those who fasted for less than thirteen hours on average every night were 36 percent more likely to see their cancer come back than women who fasted for thirteen hours or more.[19] Thus, using nightly fasting periods of more than thirteen hours, plus periodic fasting-mimicking diet, plus the Longevity Diet between fasting-mimicking-diet cycles (all of which allows patients to maintain healthy but low blood glucose, insulin, and IGF-1 levels as well as a healthy weight) is expected to be beneficial against cancer's survival and metastasis—extending survival and potentially increasing remission.

Although we don't know the ideal glucose level, based on the data above we can speculate that maintaining a fasting glucose level around 70 mg/dl may be both safe and effective against cancer. But it's not a simple number to reach and maintain for the majority of patients. It may be shown in future studies that lower glucose levels are more beneficial, but because we also have to worry about nourishment and frailty of the patient, the 70 mg/dl target is recommended. Notably, it is possible that very low glucose levels could have negative effects on populations of immune cells that fight cancer cells.

Here is a summary of the daily diet and physical activity recommended during cancer treatment in between cycles of therapy (aside from the fasting-mimicking diet, to be discussed with your oncologist):

1. The Longevity Diet (see chapter 3 and my book *The Longevity Diet*)
2. Sugar and refined carbohydrate restriction
3. Low but sufficient proteins (0.7–0.8 grams per kilogram per day or 0.31–0.36 grams per pound per day of fish or plant proteins)—can be increased slightly if muscle mass or function drops
4. A 13- to 14–hour overnight fast
5. Exercise and strength training (see chapter 3)

OTHER NUTRITIONAL THERAPIES IN BREAST CANCER TREATMENT: THE KETOGENIC DIET

A ketogenic diet is a normal-calorie, high-fat, and very low-carbohydrate regimen. Traditionally, it has been used for treating refractory epilepsy, a type of epilepsy that resists drug treatments,[20] in children. The ratio among macronutrients is four parts fats to one part carbs and proteins.

Ketogenic diets represent an emerging complementary strategy for managing cancer. However, most of the clinical trials using the ketogenic diet have focused on brain tumors. The initial clinical studies indicate that the ketogenic diet likely has no substantial therapeutic activity when used as single agent in patients with cancer and that the potential benefits of this diet should be sought in combination with other conventional approaches depending on the tumor type/subtype, such as chemotherapy, radiotherapy, antiangiogenic treatments (reducing the growth of new blood vessels),

PI3K inhibitors (drugs that inhibit those enzymes that are part of signaling pathways for cellular growth and metabolism), and fasting or the fasting-mimicking diet.[21]

In regard to the ketogenic diet and breast cancer, I will focus on the effect of a ketogenic diet in breast cancer patients with or without metastases. In a randomized and controlled trial, sixty patients with locally advanced or metastatic breast cancer and planned chemotherapy were asked to follow either a ketogenic (experimental group) or a standard (control group) diet for three months. Women following the ketogenic diet had a decrease in fasting blood sugar, weight, and body fat percentage, with no severe adverse side effect.[22] In another study of eighty patients undergoing treatment with chemotherapy, forty were assigned a ketogenic diet while the other forty were assigned a standard diet for twelve weeks. The results showed a decrease in inflammatory markers, insulin, and tumor size in those following the ketogenic diet.[23]

Despite the promising results of the ketogenic diet, there are no conclusive data about its efficacy against cancer progression in patients, although it may reduce blood glucose and IGF-1. A major concern is that ketogenic diets are in most cases not plant-based, so

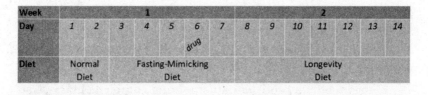

Week	1							2						
Day	1	2	3	4	5	6	7	8	9	10	11	12	13	14
						drug								
Diet	Normal Diet			Fasting-Mimicking Diet						Longevity Diet				

Week	3							4						
Day	15	16	17	18	19	20	21	22	23	24	25	26	27	28
Diet	Longevity Diet							Ketogenic Diet						

4.17. *This is an example of a four-week diet regimen combined with a very aggressive treatment for a cancer that doesn't respond to standard therapies; this should be personalized by an experienced team or as part of a clinical trial. In this case, the patient is receiving cancer treatment every four weeks combined with a fasting-mimicking diet, followed by two weeks of the Longevity Diet, one week of a ketogenic diet, and two days of a normal diet, while monitoring weight, muscle mass, blood markers, and cancer progression.*

they contain high levels of animal proteins, which could accelerate the progression of certain cancers. In cases of advanced and incurable cancer and if new and positive clinical studies support it, patients should talk to their oncologist and a nutritionist about following a plant-based and relatively low-protein ketogenic diet while focusing on maintaining muscle mass and avoiding malnourishment. Patients who decide to adopt a ketogenic diet can alternate this diet with a periodic fasting-mimicking diet and the Longevity Diet, which our clinics have applied to a number of patients, especially glioma patients (figure 4.17).[24] Below is an example of a very aggressive treatment combining various strategies.

PATIENTS' STORIES AND EXPERIENCES

Nora Quinn, California

Nora was diagnosed with breast cancer in the spring of 2009. What was originally thought to be a cyst turned out to be a malignant and very aggressive triple-negative tumor breast cancer, stage I. She had two surgeries and several radiotherapy treatments. Before she was scheduled to start chemotherapy, she found an article describing one of our studies on breast cancer in mice in the *Los Angeles Times*.

One group of mice was treated with chemotherapy, while mice in the other group were fasted for two days before being given chemotherapy. Nora recalled, "The difference in survival rates was startling. Only a small number of mice in the group who simply received chemotherapy survived, while in the second group, nearly all of the mice survived. Those mice in the first group all lost some hair, while the mice in the second group did not lose any hair. I remember thinking, *Well, I know which group I want to be in.*"

She recounted that none of her doctors said anything to her about the impact of nutrition on breast cancer; on the contrary, every single medical office she went to had a bowl of candy on the check-in counter, and most of the staff was overweight. She decided to undergo two seven-day water-fasting periods (which I did not advise).

She wrote: "My first chemotherapy treatment was July 3, 2009. As I walked to the infusion room, I saw a table covered with 4th of July frosted cupcakes, cookies, brownies, muffins, and candy for the patients and staff. There was not a single piece of any food that could be called healthy on that table. I asked a staff member why all the food was just sweets and she said, 'Oh, we just want to get calories into them, because they have cancer.' This seemed crazy to me. I had four chemotherapy treatments. There was always a table of pastries available for patients."

A couple of years after having breast cancer, she joined a clinical trial at USC that tested the fasting-mimicking diet in healthy patients. After the study was concluded, she tried to continue periods of five hundred calories a day but never felt quite as good as she had during the study, eating the food provided there. "I was very pleased to hear that the five-day fasting-mimicking diet program is available for the public," she wrote later. "I have now used it many times. It is difficult at first, but I find that if as I fall asleep, I remind myself what I will be eating the next day, it is much easier. I always feel refreshed after the program."

As of 2023, her breast cancer has not returned. A few years ago, a mammogram showed a lesion on the opposite breast, and she was told to immediately get an ultrasound. She went home and did a seven-day fast. Then she had the ultrasound. The lesion was gone. "I feel very fortunate to have discovered the work of Dr. Longo," she says.

Christopher Gregg, PhD, Associate Professor of Neurobiology and Human Genetics, University of Utah

Christopher is a scientist with stage IV breast cancer, meaning the cancer has spread to other parts of his body. Over the past few years, he has followed my advice to integrate the fasting-mimicking diet into his treatment.

He used a combination of the fasting-mimicking diet or forty-eight-hour water fasting with every infusion treatment and restricted eating (10:00 a.m.–6:00 p.m.). Christopher had metastatic disease throughout his bones, spine, hips, and femur when we began. After seven months of chemotherapy and fasting, he reached NED (no evidence of disease) by scans and tumor markers. This is an unusual outcome but consistent with what we saw in patients who were enrolled in clinical trials. As of now, he remains in remission and continues to follow the fasting-mimicking diet every three months, forty-eight-hour water fasting every month or more, and restricted eating five days per week.

BREAST CANCER TREATMENT SUMMARY

- Follow oncologist recommendations and standard-of-care therapy (surgery, radiotherapy, immunotherapy, chemotherapy, kinase inhibitors, etc.) based on the specific stage and biology of your cancer.
- Talk to your oncologist about combining the standard therapy with a fasting-mimicking diet.
- Unless discouraged by your oncologist and dietitian for specific reasons, fast for thirteen to fourteen hours a day (for example, eating only between 8:00 a.m. and 6:00 p.m.) during therapy.
- Between treatments maintain a Longevity Diet.
- If the therapy combinations described in this chapter are not sufficient, talk to your oncologist and a nutrition healthcare professional to alternate the fasting-mimicking diet and the Longevity Diet with a low-protein and plant-and-fish-based ketogenic diet, making sure it does not negatively affect your body mass or immune system.
- Maintain a normal body weight.
- Be physically active and exercise, after consulting your oncologist.

- Try to keep your phase angle (an indicator of muscular function) above 5 by working on muscle strength at least three or four times a week for thirty to forty minutes; you can follow the exercise video on the Create Cures website's section "Exercise and Longevity."

Patients who would like to learn more about the fasting/nutrition-based interventions described in this chapter should contact the Longevity and Healthspan Clinic of the Create Cures Foundation.

5

FASTING, NUTRITION, AND GYNECOLOGICAL CANCERS

For their contributions and revisions to this chapter, I thank Giuseppe Curigliano, MD, head of the Division of Early Drug Development at the European Institute of Oncology, IRCCS, in Milan, and associate professor of medical oncology at the University of Milan; Alessandro Laviano, MD, associate professor of medicine in the Department of Translational and Precision Medicine at Sapienza University of Rome; Andreas Michalsen, MD, professor of integrative medicine at the Institute of Social Medicine, Epidemiology, and Health Economics of the Charité University Medical Center in Berlin and director of the Department of Internal and Integrative Medicine at the Immanuel Hospital in Berlin; and Hanno Pijl, MD, internist-endocrinologist in the Department of Internal Medicine of the Leiden University Medical Center in the Netherlands and professor of diabetology at Leiden University.

GYNECOLOGICAL CANCERS:
WHAT THEY ARE AND HOW THEY ARE TREATED

Each year, about 94,000 women in the U.S. are diagnosed with gynecological cancers, which include all malignancies involving a woman's reproductive organs and genitals. The five major types of gynecological cancers are ovarian, cervical, endometrial (uterine), vaginal, and vulvar.[1]

1. There were nearly 314,000 new cases of ovarian cancer globally in 2020.[2]

2. Cervical tumors are among the most frequent gynecological cancers in the world, with more than 600,000 new cases in 2020.[3]

3. Endometrial (uterine) cancer is the most common gynecological cancer in developed countries, with an increasing incidence, up from 320,000 new cases in 2012 to more than 417,000 new cases in 2020 globally.[4]

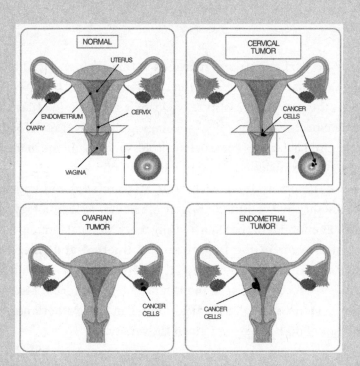

5.1. *Cancers of the ovaries, cervix, and endometrium are the most common types of gynecological cancers. Ovarian cancer originates from the surface of the ovary. Endometrial cancer begins in the layer of cells that form the lining (endometrium) of the uterus. Cervical cancer occurs in the cells of the cervix, the lower part of the uterus that connects to the vagina.*

OVARIAN CANCER AND TREATMENT

Ovarian cancer affects women of all ages, with greater frequency between fifty and sixty-five years of age. Even if it has a relatively low incidence, ovarian cancer can be very aggressive, probably due to the fact that it often does not cause recognizable symptoms in the early stages, making it difficult to diagnose until advanced stages.

Among the main risk factors for ovarian cancer in women are nulliparity (never having given birth), a first pregnancy after thirty-five years of age, hormone replacement therapy, early menarche (menstrual cycle), and late menopause. On the other hand, protective factors are pregnancy before the age of twenty-five, a high number of pregnancies, use of oral contraceptives, and breastfeeding.

Ovarian cancers are classified in different categories based on the cells from which they originate, with 90 percent of malignant tumors coming from epithelial cells (epithelial ovarian cancer, or EOC) in the lining that covers the outer surface of the ovary.

Surgery is key in the management of ovarian cancer, and it is performed based on the type and stage of the tumor. For example, in the case of advanced ovarian cancer, the goal of surgery is to remove all of the macroscopically visible tumor. This result, when obtained, improves the prognosis, and favors the effect of chemotherapy.

After surgery, the standard of care for ovarian cancer are cycles of chemotherapy or a more targeted therapy.[5]

CERVICAL CANCER AND TREATMENT

The main risk factor for cervical cancer is human papillomavirus (HPV), a common asymptomatic infection, mainly transmitted by sexual contact, that usually resolves itself quickly. Around 75 percent of women contract it at least once in their lifetimes. Sometimes it can cause abnormal tissue growth, such as warts, and other cellular changes. These benign changes can become tumors if left untreated, although it can take twenty to thirty years to develop. Thus, tumors diagnosed in forty-five- or fifty-year-old women could be the result of infections contracted in their teens or twenties. Other risk factors, albeit to a much lesser extent than papillomavirus, are cigarette smoking and sexually transmitted diseases (chlamydial infections, herpes, etc.).

The good news is that cervical cancer is an increasingly preventable disease, because a vaccine can prevent papillomavirus infection and there are screening tests, such as the HPV test and Pap test, that can detect the infection caused by the papillomavirus in the early stages.

The therapies, which vary according to the degree of invasion of the tumor and the patient's age, include surgery, chemotherapy, and radiotherapy, as well as immunotherapy for metastatic tumors.

ENDOMETRIAL CANCER AND TREATMENT

The menstrual cycle involves a natural shedding of the endometrium, the inner layer of the uterus, which is a protective factor against endometrial cancer for women who still menstruate. Because of this, it is diagnosed more prevalently in postmenopausal women. Obesity and type 2 diabetes are also well-established risk factors for this tumor. Since endometrial cancer exhibits several symptoms (for example, abnormal bleeding in menopausal women), cancer is often diagnosed early, when the tumor is still limited to the uterine body. For this reason, the chance of successful treatment and remission is often good.

Conservative therapy for endometrial cancer is based on the use of hormones with progestogens (steroid hormones) to promote cancer cell death and restore normalcy to the endometrium.[6]

FASTING AND THE FASTING-MIMICKING DIET IN GYNECOLOGICAL CANCER TREATMENT

Laboratory Research

In our 2012 mouse study, we tested the effects of fasting on a number of different cancer types, including ovarian cancer. We were able to show that whereas the cycles of fasting alone did not slow down the growth of human ovarian cancer cells, either chemotherapy or the combination of fasting cycles and chemotherapy were effective in preventing cancer growth.[7]

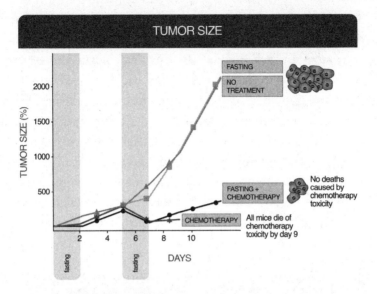

5.2. *In mice, fasting cycles alone did not slow cancer growth, while chemotherapy or the combination of fasting cycles and chemotherapy were effective in preventing the growth of human ovarian cancer cells. However, all mice treated with chemotherapy alone died early from the therapy's side effects. Modified from Changhan Lee et al., "Fasting Cycles Retard Growth of Tumors and Sensitize a Range of Cancer Cell Types to Chemotherapy,"* Science Translational Medicine *4, no. 124 (2012): 124ra27.*

However, in the absence of the fasting cycles, chemotherapy's side effects caused early death in the mice. The combination of fasting and chemotherapy was able to prevent both cancer growth and the toxicity of chemotherapy (figure 5.2).

Based on our studies with many other cancer types in both mice and humans, it is likely that the combination of a number of therapies aimed at treating ovarian cancer with the fasting-mimicking diet would be more effective against the cancer than just standard therapies alone. Thus, fasting-mimicking-diet cycles are expected to not only reduce the toxicity of the standard cancer treatment but also increase its effectiveness. However, large, randomized clinical trials focused on gynecological cancers and the fasting / fasting-mimicking diet will be necessary to determine if this dietary intervention improves the effects of the cancer therapy in humans as it does in mice.

In 2020, we completed a mouse study in which we tested tamoxifen plus the fasting-mimicking diet and gynecological side effects. Tamoxifen, a hormonal therapy that blocks the action of estrogen in breast cancer patients, can cause excessive endometrial growth. We showed that fasting-mimicking-diet cycles not only reduced endometrial growth and uterus weight in mice treated with tamoxifen but also had the same effect in untreated mice, raising the possibility that it has the potential to reduce endometrial growth (figure 5.3), a risk factor for uterine cancer, in women who do not have cancer. For these reasons, it will be important to study the effects of fasting-mimicking-diet cycles in

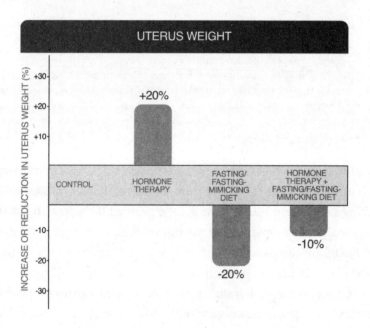

5.3. *Tamoxifen hormone therapy, in addition to blocking the action of estrogen in mice with breast cancer, causes excessive growth leading to increased endometrium weight. This is a risk factor for uterine cancer. Fasting / fasting-mimicking-diet cycles not only reduced uterus weight and endometrial growth in mice treated with tamoxifen but also had the same effect in untreated mice. Modified from Irene Caffa et al., "Fasting-Mimicking Diet and Hormone Therapy Induce Breast Cancer Regression,"* Nature *583, no. 7817 (2020): 620–24.*

combination with standard therapies in women who suffer from any gynecological cancer, as well as those experiencing abnormal endometrial growth.[8]

GYNECOLOGICAL CANCER, FASTING, AND FASTING-MIMICKING DIET: CLINICAL STUDIES

Although the use of fasting / fasting-mimicking diets in the treatment of patients with gynecological cancers is in its initial stages, here we present both case reports and clinical studies on this topic.

Case Reports from Gynecology Clinics

Before publishing our first paper on the effect of fasting on cancer treatment in mice in 2008,[9] I, together with Fernando Safdie, a medical doctor working in my laboratory at USC in Los Angeles, started to collect data from oncologists treating patients who were fasting in combination with cancer treatment (in most cases, chemotherapy). Out of the ten patients who were included in the first clinical report on fasting and cancer, two were women with gynecological cancers: uterine and ovarian.[10]

PATIENT 1: 74-YEAR-OLD FEMALE, STAGE IV UTERINE CANCER

- During the first chemotherapy cycle, the patient had a normal diet and reported fatigue, weakness, hair loss, headache, and gastrointestinal discomfort.
- In cycles two through six, the patient fasted in combination with chemotherapy and reported a reduction in the side effects (figure 5.4).

The patient fasted:

1. for thirty-six hours before carboplatin + paclitaxel chemotherapy on her second cycle of chemotherapy;
2. for sixty hours before carboplatin + paclitaxel chemotherapy on cycles three and four; and
3. for sixty hours prior to and twenty-four hours after the same chemotherapy on cycles five and six.

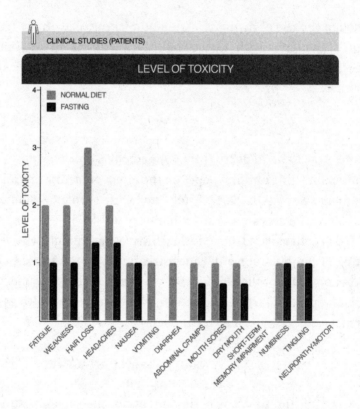

5.4. *The reported side effects of chemotherapy in a seventy-four-year-old patient with stage IV uterine cancer (meaning the metastatic tumor had reached the bladder or intestine) were generally higher during the cycle of chemotherapy when she did not fast (gray bars) than during subsequent cycles when the patient fasted in combination with chemotherapy (black bars). In some cases, side effects seem to be absent (for example, vomiting, diarrhea, and impairment of short-term memory). Toxicity levels range from 0 (no toxicity) to 4 (high toxicity). Modified from Fernando M. Safdie et al., "Fasting and Cancer Treatment in Humans: A Case Series Report," Aging 1, no. 12 (2009): 988–1007.*

The results after fasting cycles along with standard therapy were an 87 percent reduction of CA 125 (cancer antigen 125), one of the key markers associated with ovarian cancer progression, and reduction in lymph node size (determined by computed tomography, CT, scan). Considering that therapy alone could have caused these effects, we do not know how much fasting contributed to the results.

PATIENT 2: 44-YEAR-OLD FEMALE, STAGE IA OVARIAN CANCER

A forty-four-year-old Caucasian female was diagnosed with a ten-by-twelve-centimeter mass in the right ovary. She had a stage IA carcinosarcoma of the ovary with no cancer detected in lymph nodes. Carcinosarcoma is a malignant cancer that is a mixture of carcinoma (cancer of epithelial tissues such as skin and tissues that cover or line the internal organs) and sarcoma (cancer of connective tissues such as bone, fat, and cartilage).

The patient's history was the following:

- She received six chemotherapy cycles consisting of ifosfamide and CDDP.
- She remained free of disease until an MRI revealed multiple new pulmonary nodules one year later. Consequently, chemotherapy with Taxol, carboplatin, and bevacizumab was initiated.
- By November, however, a CT scan showed progression of the cancer.
- Treatment was changed to gemcitabine chemotherapy plus Taxol, complemented with G-CSF (Neulasta), which is a medicine that stimulates the growth of white blood cells and reduces the risk of infection.
- After the first dose of gemcitabine (900 mg/m^2), the patient experienced prolonged neutropenia—an abnormally low number of a type of white blood cells called neutrophils, which increases the risk of infection. She also had

developed thrombocytopenia, a condition in which the number of platelets (thrombocytes)—important in helping blood to clot—is low. These two conditions forced a delay in the treatment.

- During the second cycle the patient received a reduced dose of gemcitabine (720 mg/m^2), but she again developed prolonged neutropenia and thrombocytopenia, causing additional treatment delays.
- For the third through sixth cycles, the patient fasted for sixty-two hours before and twenty-four hours after chemotherapy.

The results after fasting cycles were added to the standard therapy were the following:

1. The patient showed a faster recovery of her blood-cell counts, allowing the completion of the chemotherapy regimen (720mg/m^2 gemcitabine on day 1, plus 720mg/m^2 gemcitabine and 80mg/m^2 Taxol on day 8).
2. During the fifth cycle, she fasted under the same regimen and received a full dose of gemcitabine (900mg/m^2) and Taxol.
3. Her blood counts (neutrophils, lymphocytes, platelets, etc.) showed consistent improvement during the cycles in which chemotherapy was combined with fasting (figure 5.5).

Notably, the improvements caused by fasting seem to be in addition to those caused by Neulasta, a drug that stimulates the growth of white blood cells, although randomized clinical trials will be necessary to test these combination therapies.

· · · · · · ·

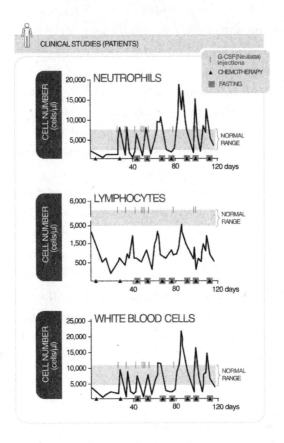

5.5. *The forty-four-year-old patient with malignant ovarian carcinosarcoma showed an improvement in her white blood cell counts, including the numbers of neutrophils (a type of white blood cell that protects against infection) and lymphocytes (another type of white blood cell that is part of the immune system), during the cycles in which the chemotherapy was combined with fasting + G-CSF (Neulasta) but not when chemotherapy and G-CSF were combined with a normal diet. Modified from Fernando M. Safdie et al., "Fasting and Cancer Treatment in Humans: A Case Series Report," Aging, 1, no. 12 (2009): 988–1007.*

CLINICAL STUDY NUMBER 1: SAFETY AND FEASIBILITY OF 24- TO 72-HOUR FASTING IN COMBINATION WITH CHEMOTHERAPY

In this clinical study done by oncologists Tanya Dorff and David Quinn in a collaboration with my group at the University of Southern California Norris Comprehensive Cancer Center in Los Angeles, twenty patients, most with gynecological or breast cancers, fasted for twenty-four, forty-eight, or seventy-two hours in combination with chemotherapy, which in most cases included gemcitabine and cisplatin. The study focused on toxicity instead of antitumor efficacy.[11]

Even though this small study was mainly aimed at determining whether fasting for one to three days could be safely combined with chemotherapy treatment, we were able to assess whether a longer fast (seventy-two hours) could be protective against multiple side effects of chemotherapy. Compared with those who fasted for twenty-four hours, the patients who fasted for seventy-two hours appeared to have reduced nausea and vomiting, as well as reduced major decreases in blood cells and reduced neuropathies, which can include numbness or pain, mostly in the hands and feet. This study also showed a reduction in the DNA damage to normal immune cells in patients who had fasted for either forty-eight or seventy-two hours compared with those who fasted for twenty-four hours (figure 5.6), in agreement with similar results in breast cancer patients.

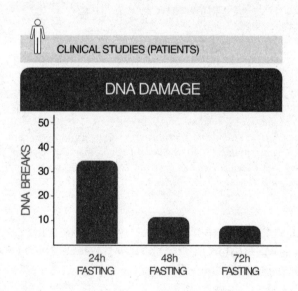

5.6. *Cancer patients who had fasted for forty-eight or seventy-two hours showed less DNA damage in normal immune cells than did patients who fasted for twenty-four hours. Modified from Tanya B. Dorff et al., "Safety and Feasibility of Fasting in Combination with Platinum-Based Chemotherapy," BMC Cancer 16 (2016).*

In many cases, however, the number of patients was too small for the trial to be statistically significant, underlining the need for larger randomized clinical trials to test these combined therapies.

CLINICAL STUDY NUMBER 2: EFFECTS OF A FASTING-MIMICKING DIET ON THE SIDE EFFECTS CAUSED BY CHEMOTHERAPY

In this clinical study by the Andreas Michalsen group and a team of oncologists at Charité Hospital in Berlin, a modified three-day fasting-mimicking diet was tested on women with either breast or ovarian cancer who were receiving chemotherapy. This trial was a randomized crossover trial, which means that patients were assigned to receive chemotherapy either with a normal diet or with a special vegan fasting-mimicking diet. After receiving three cycles of chemotherapy, those on the fasting diet resumed a normal diet and those on the normal diet started a fasting-mimicking diet.

The thirty-four patients who completed the trial reported a reduction in side effects and improvements in their quality of life when they combined chemotherapy with the modified fasting-mimicking diet compared with when chemotherapy was combined with a normal diet.

CLINICAL STUDY NUMBERS 3 AND 4: FASTING AND ITS EFFECT ON CHEMOTHERAPY ADMINISTRATION IN GYNECOLOGICAL TUMORS

The first study was carried out on twenty patients: eleven with ovarian cancer, eight with uterine cancer, and one with cervical cancer. Ninety percent received taxane and platinum-based chemotherapy. Patients were asked to fast for twenty-four hours before and twenty-four hours after each chemotherapy cycle. The women received at least six planned chemotherapy cycles combined with fasting or with their regular diet.[12]

The results showed that short-term fasting was safe in combination with chemotherapy in gynecological cancer patients without

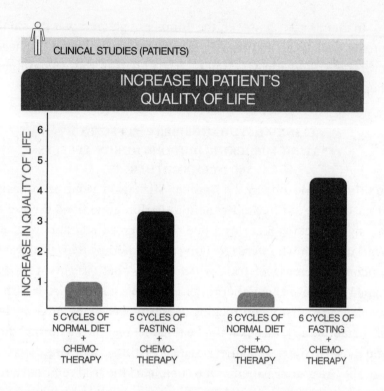

CLINICAL STUDIES (PATIENTS)

INCREASE IN PATIENT'S QUALITY OF LIFE

5.7. *The quality of life of patients who followed fasting in combination with chemotherapy improved over the course of treatment (black bars) while those on a normal diet (gray bars) did not see improvement. Modified from Courtney J. Riedinger et al., "Water Only Fasting and Its Effect on Chemotherapy Administration in Gynecologic Malignancies," Gynecologic Oncology 159, no. 3 (December 2020): 799–803.*

significant toxicity or weight loss; the quality of life of the patients who fasted in combination with chemotherapy improved over the course of treatment (figure 5.7); and those who fasted required fewer reductions in the dose of chemotherapy or delays in the scheduled treatment (figure 5.8).

Notably, in the half of patients who combined fasting with chemotherapy, none showed cancer progression, whereas 20 percent of the patients who were on a normal diet saw their tumors progress (figure 5.9).

A 2020 article published in *BMC Cancer* showed that a four-day very-low-calorie fast during chemotherapy can increase patients'

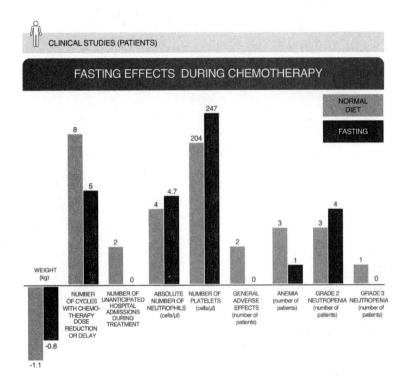

5.8. *Patients who followed fasting in combination with chemotherapy showed (1) less weight reduction; (2) fewer delayed or reduced chemotherapy cycles; (3) no unexpected hospitalization; (4) an increase in blood cells (neutrophils, i.e., white blood cells important for the immune system, and platelets, blood cells that help the blood clot); (5) few to no serious side effects; (6) less anemia; and (7) less grade 3 (more severe) neutropenia, but a slightly higher rate of grade 2 (less severe) neutropenia. Modified from Courtney J. Riedinger et al., "Water Only Fasting and Its Effect on Chemotherapy Administration in Gynecologic Malignancies,"* Gynecologic Oncology, *159, no. 3 (2020): 799–803.*

tolerance to the chemotherapy and reduce its toxicity, in agreement with the studies described above. These are the results of a cross-pilot study conducted on thirty patients: twenty-two with breast cancer, two with endometrial cancer, two with ovarian cancer, and four with cervical cancer.[13]

During half of the chemotherapy cycles the patients fasted for ninety-six hours (with a maximum of four hundred to six hundred calories per day), and during the other half they ate normally.

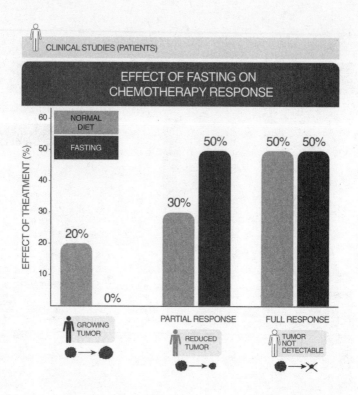

5.9. Among the ten patients who fasted during chemotherapy, (1) none showed disease progression; (2) 50 percent showed a reduction in tumor size; and (3) 50 percent showed a complete regression of the tumor. On the other hand, among the ten patients who ate a normal diet during chemotherapy, (1) 20 percent showed disease progression; (2) 30 percent showed a reduction in tumor size; and (3) 50 percent showed a complete regression of the tumor. Modified from Courtney J. Riedinger et al., "Water Only Fasting and Its Effect on Chemotherapy Administration in Gynecologic Malignancies," Gynecologic Oncology *159, no. 3 (2020): 799–803.*

Modified fasting ninety-six hours before chemotherapy improved its tolerability. Patients who fasted reported a reduction in side effects, such as less inflammation in the mouth (stomatitis), headache, and general weakness, confirming that this protocol is safe, is well tolerated, and may have a protective effect. In addition, patients who fasted saw a reduction in average body weight and in insulin and IGF-1, without altering normal blood counts.

Since fasting can be hard to sustain, the researchers decided to test the ketogenic diet, given that fasting and the ketogenic diet can cause some overlapping changes, including the production of ketone bodies (used as a source of energy during fasting). So the study also had half of the patients follow the ketogenic diet for six days before each fasting period to see if it could be useful to reduce the discomfort of fasting. But the study showed the ketogenic diet did not decrease the discomfort associated with the latter, nor did it increase adherence by patients. In fact, patients found it more difficult to practice the ketogenic diet before fasting than just to fast. Added to this is the fact that the ketogenic diet, when compared with fasting, did not cause beneficial effects on chemotherapy-induced toxicity or on other parameters taken into account by this study.[14]

IN SUMMARY, AT LEAST FOUR explorative clinical studies and two case reports including patients with a variety of gynecological cancers have monitored patients receiving chemotherapy in combination with fasting or the fasting-mimicking diet. Although these studies are small, together they suggest that fasting-mimicking diets are safe in combination with a variety of chemotherapy drugs. They also provide initial evidence that fasting and the fasting-mimicking diet can reduce side effects ranging from nausea and vomiting to reduced blood-cell counts to DNA damage in normal cells, possibly preventing drug dose reduction or delays of therapy and, in some cases, patients' hospitalization. Furthermore, the preliminary evidence points to better quality of life during chemotherapy when undergoing a fasting-mimicking diet.

Most of the major research centers around the world, including ours, that are studying fasting and cancer treatment have moved away from water-only fasting and have endorsed the use of the fasting-mimicking diet, which is safer, since it allows patients to consume food daily, thus increasing the ability of patients to remain on the diet compared with water-only fasting. The use of the fasting-mimicking diet will also be essential in allowing fasting to become a standardized therapy regulated by or at least following the standards of the FDA in the U.S. and other regulatory agencies around the world.

These results, together with the larger randomized clinical trials on breast cancer presented in the previous chapter, indicate that fasting-mimicking diets have the potential to improve gynecological cancer therapy.

Although the fasting-mimicking diet appears to be the most promising and feasible dietary treatment in combination with standard drugs, it is also important to examine and discuss other nutritional therapies that have been used in support of gynecological cancer drugs, particularly the ketogenic diet.

EVERYDAY NUTRITION, INCLUDING KETOGENIC DIET, IN GYNECOLOGICAL CANCER THERAPY

A systematic review published in 2015 in the journal *Gynecologic Oncology* by English and Dutch researchers analyzed eight different studies with 255 endometrial cancer survivors and 122 ovarian cancer survivors. Data suggest that both exercise and dietary interventions should be encouraged to achieve weight loss, when needed, and improvement in physical fitness.[15]

In a more recent randomized, controlled trial, published in 2018, women with ovarian or endometrial cancer were assigned to a ketogenic diet, which entailed a significant reduction in carbohydrate intake (only 5 percent of the typical calorie intake) or the American Cancer Society (ACS) diet, with high fiber intake and low fat intake, for twelve weeks. In comparison with the ACS diet, women following the ketogenic diet showed lower levels of total and visceral fat and insulin. Because visceral fat can produce pro-inflammatory molecules that can promote the proliferation of cancer cells, its reduction may be a factor that contributes to a decrease in the growth of tumors.[16]

In a following paper, the same research group evaluated the

effects of the two diets on physical and mental health status, hunger or satiety, and food cravings in women with ovarian or endometrial cancer through questionnaires. The data showed that a ketogenic diet did not negatively affect quality of life. On the contrary, it improved physical function, increased energy, and diminished specific food cravings, even if patients following the ketogenic diet consumed significantly fewer calories than the subjects on the control diet. This can, in turn, suggest that some of the effects could be ascribed to the lower energy intake.[17]

To ensure the best outcome, an experienced physician in integrative medicine and/or an experienced dietitian or nutritionist should be involved to help the patient correctly combine the ketogenic diet (which should be as plant-based as possible), the fasting-mimicking diet, and the Longevity Diet without losing muscle mass or function.

In conclusion, fasting-mimicking diets and other nutritional interventions can be effective tools to support cancer treatments, but further research is needed to test and understand their full potential.

GYNECOLOGICAL CANCER TREATMENT SUMMARY

- Follow standard cancer therapy (chemotherapy, immunotherapy, kinase inhibitors, etc.).
- Talk to your oncologist about combining it with a fasting-mimicking diet.
- Between treatments, follow the Longevity Diet (see chapter 3).
- Fast for thirteen to fourteen hours a day (for example, eat from 8:00 a.m. to 6:00 p.m.).
- Maintain a healthy body weight.
- After consulting with an oncologist, be physically active and exercise.

- Try to keep your phase angle (an indicator of muscular function) above 5 by working on muscle strength at least three or four times a week for thirty to forty minutes; you can follow the exercise video on the Create Cures website's section "Exercise and Longevity."

Patients who would like to learn more about the fasting/nutrition-based interventions described in this chapter should contact the Longevity and Healthspan Clinic of the Create Cures Foundation.

6

FASTING, NUTRITION, AND PROSTATE CANCER

For their contributions to and revisions of this chapter, I would like to thank Frank Sullivan, MD, medical director of the Oncology Radiation Department of the Galway Clinic, founding director of the Prostate Cancer Institute (PCI), and adjunct professor of medicine at the National University of Ireland in Galway; David Quinn, MD, medical director of the Norris Cancer Hospital and Clinics, head of the Section of Genitourinary Medical Oncology and associate professor of medicine in the Division of Cancer Medicine and Blood Diseases at the Keck School of Medicine of USC; Tanya Dorff, MD, oncologist and professor in the Department of Medical Oncology & Therapeutics Research at the City of Hope Medical Clinic in Duarte, California; Alessandro Laviano, MD, associate professor of medicine in the Department of Translational and Precision Medicine at Sapienza University in Rome; Hanno Pijl, MD, internist-endocrinologist in the Department of Internal Medicine at the Leiden University Medical Center in the Netherlands and professor of diabetology at the University of Leiden.

PROSTATE CANCER: WHAT IT IS AND HOW IT IS TREATED

Prostate cancer is the second-most-common cancer in men and the fourth-most-common cancer overall, with 1.4 million new cases in 2020 worldwide.[1] In the last twenty-five years the number of diagnoses has risen, in part due to the general aging of the population and the introduction of prostate-specific antigen (PSA)–based screening, leading to increased detection in asymptomatic patients and earlier diagnoses.

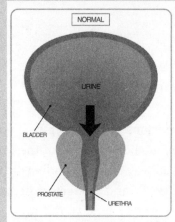 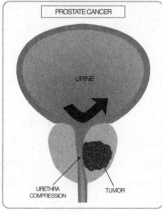

6.1. *The prostate gland is located just below the bladder in men and surrounds the top of the urethra, the tube that drains urine from the bladder. Under normal conditions, the prostate is the size of a walnut, while in the presence of cancer the central portion of the prostate swells and the overgrowth of this tissue compresses the urethra, creating problems in the passage of urine.*

As is the case for other tumors, prostate cancer incidence is affected by both genetic risk factors (first-degree relative with prostate or other cancer) and environmental factors, such as pollution. Other risk factors for prostate cancer include

1. age (it rarely occurs under the age of forty-five);

2. race (it is more common in African American and Afro Caribbean men);

3. selected germ-line mutations (such as DNA-repair defects and mismatch repair genes);

4. hormonal factors such as exogenous androgen consumption and IGF-1; and

5. overall health factors, including diet (the risk increases with a high intake of fat, meat, and calcium) and exercise.

In most cases, prostate cancer grows very slowly, so often men will die of other causes before the cancer becomes life-threatening. Nutrition can be particularly important for its prevention and also for its treatment. As previously observed, the best approach is not to focus on the prevention of a particular cancer or disease but rather to adopt a lifestyle designed to extend healthy longevity, like the Longevity Diet, unless there are risk factors for prostate cancer.

The most common diagnostic technique for prostate cancer is a screening biomarker (PSA) in a patient who is either asymptomatic or complaining of lower-urinary-tract symptoms (frequency, urgency, discomfort urinating, etc.). If the PSA level is high, then prostate imaging (MRI) and a biopsy (tissue sampling) will be needed. If a diagnosis of prostate cancer is established by a biopsy, a further series of diagnostic scans may be needed to establish the stage of the disease to help guide the treatment options. Such options are highly dependent on several factors and are best decided by a multidisciplinary clinical team. Irrespective of the treatment option chosen, patient outcomes are highly dependent on the following:

1. Overall health and presence or absence of other diseases.

2. The clinical stage—in other words, the size and precise location of the cancer in the body at time of treatment.

3. The cancer's grade, as determined by assessment from a biopsy or surgery. The Gleason grading system is the commonly used system.[2]

4. Age and life expectancy, since in some cases the treatments carry such a high risk of serious side effects that the oncologist needs to decide whether a particular therapy is appropriate or not considering the age of the patient and how long he/she is otherwise expected to live.

Treatment options for prostate cancer can be *curative* (for early-stage or locally confined cancers) or focused on *containment*, for later stages or patients with widespread (metastatic) or recurrent disease.

There are several options for patients with locally confined or early-stage disease, which typically involve either surgery (radical prostatectomy) or radiation (external beam or implanted radiation brachytherapy) or a combination of both. Because prostate cancer cells use testosterone to fuel growth, hormone therapy is often utilized to decrease testicular testosterone production, often in conjunction with radiation. In widespread disease, the mainstay of treatment is a systemic/drug treatment. This can include androgen-deprivation therapy (ADT), which reduces the levels of activity of testosterone, as well as chemotherapy (e.g., docetaxel, cabazitaxel, etc.).

Radiation treatment may be combined with androgen-deprivation therapy, which can be continued for several months after the radiation treatment.

Since a full discussion of all the factors is beyond the scope of this chapter, patients, along with their families, should discuss with their team what is best for them, given that the therapies can have side effects and can significantly affect quality of life.

Although hormone therapy can be initially highly effective for almost all patients, inevitably cancer cells become resistant to this therapy. At this stage, treatment may include immunotherapy (for example, sipuleucel-T), advanced androgen-targeted therapy (oral drugs such as abiraterone or enzalutamide), or radiopharmaceutical therapy (such as radium-223), each of which blocks testosterone production and function.

Regular screening, such as measuring PSA (prostate-specific antigen) levels in the blood, is important for men over fifty, or earlier if they are at higher risk of prostate cancer based on family history and racial background.[3]

"ALTERNATIVE"
VERSUS CONVENTIONAL THERAPIES

In our many years of medical research, we have either defended integrative therapies like fasting or fasting-mimicking diet with physicians or defended standard treatments like hormone therapy or even chemotherapy with patients seeking alternative options. Doctors, especially in Western societies, have been taught to follow hospital-based procedures and adopt "evidence-based" standards of care, whereas patients often are so desperate (rightfully so) for a solution that they will turn to alternative therapies, rather than science and clinical data, to guide their decisions. They tend to rely more on word of mouth and anecdotal evidence, rather than qualitative and quantitative studies designed to answer clinical questions. Health care is complex and changes rapidly, and each treatment—either standard or alternative—alone is often not sufficient to deal with a patient who has an advanced, complex, chronic disease like metastatic cancer.

Advanced and metastatic prostate cancer is no exception. For this reason, I will make the case for combining the "fasting-mimicking-diet wild card" with existing standard therapies, including hormone therapy, chemotherapy, and radiation, to treat prostate cancer more effectively and improve patients' outcomes and quality of life. As usual, we begin with mouse studies.

LABORATORY STUDIES

In 2007, the laboratory of Vernon Steele at the National Cancer Institute in Bethesda, Maryland, used a combination of toxins and testosterone to cause prostate cancer. Then they gave the rats a normal diet or a diet that was either 15 percent or 30 percent calorie restricted (the diets were identical but less food was given to the rats). Of the rats in the study, 74 percent on the normal diet developed prostate cancer, versus 64 percent of those eating a 15 percent calorie-restricted diet and 72 percent of those eating a 30 percent calorie-restricted diet. This and other results led the authors to conclude that calorie restriction does not prevent prostate cancer.[4]

Another study, by Melissa Bonorden and her collaborators, confirmed that continuous calorie restriction did not delay prostate cancer growth or the survival of mice, whereas alternating weeks on calorie restriction with weeks of a normal calorie diet caused a minor delay in prostate cancer growth and a small increase in survival.[5] Another study in mice undergoing either continuous calorie restriction or one or two days a week of fasting also showed no effects on prostate cancer.[6]

Many of you may wonder whether I am suggesting that calorie restriction and fasting don't work against prostate cancer. Yes and no. These results are not surprising, and they are consistent with the results presented in the earlier chapters on breast and ovarian cancers. They also underline the need to understand cancer in depth, as well as the relationship between nutrients, genes, cancer cells, and cancer drugs, before one is able to prevent or successfully treat cancer. This means integrating the much more restricted fasting-mimicking diet instead of 20 to 30 percent calorie restriction, and using fasting-mimicking diets together with treatments that either exploit the weakness of starved cancer cells (chemotherapy, radiotherapy, hormone therapy) or block the starvation escape pathways activated in response to fasting-mimicking diets described in the breast cancer chapter.

In fact, in the breast cancer chapter I showed that fasting-mimicking-diet cycles alone had only a minor effect on the progression of breast cancer in mice, but they actually caused cancer regression when combined with hormone therapy and the drug palbociclib or with other drugs. Although we have not yet published our animal studies on prostate cancer, it shares a number of similarities with breast cancer. They both derive from epithelial cells and are regulated by sex hormones.[7] As described in chapter 4, most breast cancers respond to the hormone estrogen, whereas most prostate cancer cells grow in response to the male sex hormones (androgens), most notably testosterone.

Animal studies that have focused only on different forms of calorie restriction and prostate cancer have not shown major upsides, suggesting that if such approaches are used, they need to be combined with more targeted conventional therapies, as we have done for the treatment of many other cancer types in both mice and humans. At the time of publication of this book, we are working on, but have yet to publish, our results using this combined approach for prostate cancer.

FASTING, THE FASTING-MIMICKING DIET, AND PROSTATE CANCER TREATMENT: CLINICAL STUDIES

Prostate cancer is one of the most promising cancers in which to study the potential beneficial effects of fasting-mimicking diets along with standard treatments already in use in oncology clinics.

Metabolic disorders, including obesity, are a side effect of using hormone therapy for prostate cancer. Therefore, the rationale for using fasting-based approaches, including the fasting-mimicking diet, is particularly compelling in this patient population, since fasting-mimicking diet cycles are well established to reduce obesity and diabetes markers. In recognition of the frequency of these metabolic effects and this potential benefit, Dr. Frank Sullivan, medical director of the Oncology Radiation Department of the Galway Clinic in Ireland, completed a clinical study using three cycles of fasting-mimicking diet in patients with prostate cancer who also showed evidence of metabolic syndrome. Most of the thirty-four enrolled patients had androgen-deprivation therapy as a part of their cancer treatment. The results show that fasting-mimicking diet cycles were tolerated well and most patients showed significant improvements in metabolic risk factors including weight, BMI, abdominal circumference, and blood pressure. This study sets the stage for larger randomized trials testing the effect of fasting-mimicking diets on prostate cancer progression in patients also receiving standard therapies.

In addition to this early pilot study, we have anecdotally observed benefits in prostate cancer patients with metastatic disease receiving standard therapy combined with fasting. The first case was that of a medical doctor with prostate cancer who came to visit us at USC.

Case 1. Metastatic Prostate Cancer

A seventy-four-year-old Caucasian man was diagnosed in 2000 with stage II prostate adenocarcinoma. At this stage, the cancer had not spread beyond the gland, so his prostate was removed. However, not all the cancer cells were removed during the surgery, and two and a half years later, the levels of PSA (a prostate cancer biomarker) rose to 1.4 ng/ml. He received several drugs that block either the production or function of testosterone and are used to prevent cancer growth. Nevertheless, their administration had to be suspended in April 2004 due to severe side effects related to testosterone deprivation. Additional therapies, including chemotherapy, also failed to control the disease. In 2007, his PSA level reached 9 ng/ml and new bone metastases were detected. Despite the chemotherapy, his PSA level continued to increase and reached 40.6 ng/ml. The cycles of chemotherapy caused side effects including fatigue, weakness, metallic taste, dizziness, forgetfulness, memory impairment, and nerve damage in the feet, which made it difficult for him to walk (figure 6.2).

After discontinuing chemotherapy, his PSA rose rapidly, suggesting cancer progression. Chemotherapy was restarted and was combined with colony-stimulating factor (G-CSF), which stimulates the growth of white blood cells. Once again, the patient suffered significant side effects. In June 2008, chemotherapy was halted, despite a reduction in his serum PSA level, because the side effects were too severe. The patient was then enrolled in a phase III clinical trial with abiraterone acetate, a hormonal second-generation drug that blocks the production of testosterone. However, this drug worked for only a short period of time and the cancer progressed, as indicated by PSA level, which increased to 20.9 ng/dl, prompting the resumption of chemotherapy and G-CSF. This time the patient opted to fast for sixty hours prior to and

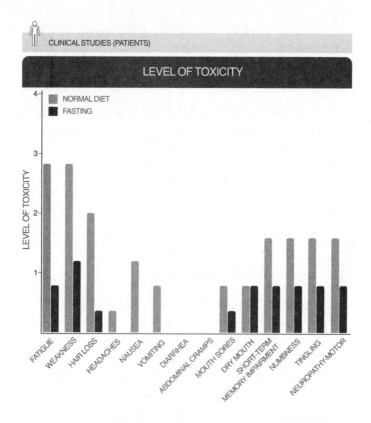

6.2. *The side effects of chemotherapy in a seventy-four-year-old man diagnosed with stage II prostate adenocarcinoma were greater during the first cycles of chemotherapy, in which he did not fast (gray bars), than during subsequent cycles in which he fasted in combination with chemotherapy (black bars). In some cases, side effects (e.g., headache, diarrhea, and abdominal pain) were absent when the patient fasted. Toxicity levels ranged from 0 (no toxicity) to 4 (high toxicity). Modified from Fernando M. Safdie et al.,* "Fasting and Cancer Treatment in Humans: A Case Series Report," Aging *1, no. 12 (2009): 988–1007.*

twenty-four hours after chemotherapy administration. Upon combining chemotherapy with fasting, the PSA level dropped, and the patient also reported considerably fewer severe side effects than in previous cycles, in which he consumed a normal diet (figure 6.2). Even after seven cycles of chemotherapy combined with fasting, the patient was able to maintain normal levels of white blood cells, including neutrophils and lymphocytes, as well as platelets, hemoglobin, and red blood cells (figure 6.3). During the last three cycles, in addition to fasting, the patient, who is a physician, in an unconventional move, applied testosterone (cream, 1 percent) for five days prior to chemotherapy. This caused a major increase in testosterone and PSA level, which reached 34.2 ng/ml. Nevertheless, three cycles of chemotherapy combined with fasting reduced PSA back to 6.43 ng/ml (figure 6.4).

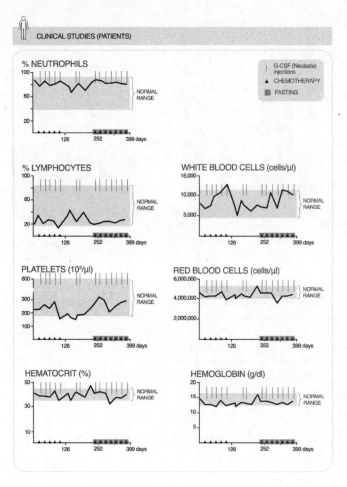

6.3. *Even after seven cycles of chemotherapy combined with fasting, the patient was able to maintain normal levels of (1) white blood cells, including neutrophils and lymphocytes, as well as (2) platelets, (3) red blood cells (which transport oxygen), (4) hemoglobin, and (5) hematocrit. Maintaining these levels is important in order to guarantee normal functioning of the immune and other blood cells. Modified from Fernando M. Safdie et al., "Fasting and Cancer Treatment in Humans: A Case Series Report,"* Aging 1, *no. 12 (2009): 988–1007.*

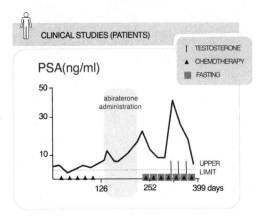

6.4. *The PSA level of a seventy-four-year-old patient with stage II prostate adenocarcinoma increased steadily even after chemotherapy and anticancer therapy (abiraterone). The PSA level dropped only with fasting cycles combined with chemotherapy. During three cycles of chemotherapy combined with fasting, the patient applied a testosterone ointment to reduce the severe side effects, which caused a significant increase in testosterone and PSA levels. However, additional cycles of chemotherapy combined with fasting reduced PSA back to 6.43 ng/ml. Modified from Fernando M. Safdie et al., "Fasting and Cancer Treatment in Humans: A Case Series Report,"* Aging, *1, no. 12 (2009): 988–1007.*

These clinical observations, along with our animal data and clinical results with other cancer types, are encouraging. They suggest that fasting and the fasting-mimicking diet could improve the tolerability and also the efficacy of hormone therapy or chemotherapy in the treatment of prostate cancer. It is possible that, when hormone therapy is combined with fasting-mimicking diet cycles and drugs blocking starvation escape pathways, this combination could cause cancer regression.

Case 2. Metastatic Prostate Cancer

This case is that of a sixty-six-year-old Caucasian male diagnosed with prostate cancer in July 1998. Initially, he presented with an early stage of the disease and was treated only with hormone therapy to block testosterone activity. In December 2000, the cancer progressed. He was placed on a second phase of hormone therapy and received radiation to the prostate and pelvis. In April 2008, a scan revealed a three-by-five-centimeter pelvic cancer mass, resulting in treatment with eight cycles of chemotherapy coupled with a growth factor to stimulate the growth of normal white blood cells. During this period the patient fasted for sixty to sixty-six hours prior to and eight to twenty-four hours following chemotherapy, with a total fast of about three days. Side effects included very mild light-headedness and a drop in blood pressure. Although the side effects of fasting were not severe, these results, as well as experiences with many other patients, convinced us to abandon the use of water-only fasting and utilize exclusively fasting-mimicking diets, which we have now shown to be associated with higher compliance and a very low level of side effects. The side effects suffered when chemotherapy was associated with fasting were minimal (figure 6.5).

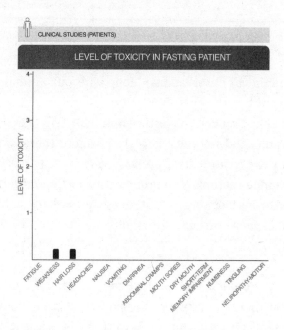

6.5. *The side effects of chemotherapy in a sixty-six-year-old man diagnosed with prostate cancer were minimal during chemotherapy in combination with fasting. In most cases side effects were absent. Toxicity levels range from 0 (no toxicity) to 4 (high toxicity). Modified from Fernando M. Safdie et al., "Fasting and Cancer Treatment in Humans: A Case Series Report,"* Aging *1, no. 12 (2009): 988–1007.*

The patient maintained normal levels of white blood cells, although he did develop anemia (low red blood cell count) (figure 6.6). His PSA level consistently decreased during the combined fasting and chemotherapy treatment, so the patient was able to return to baseline hormone therapy (figure 6.7).

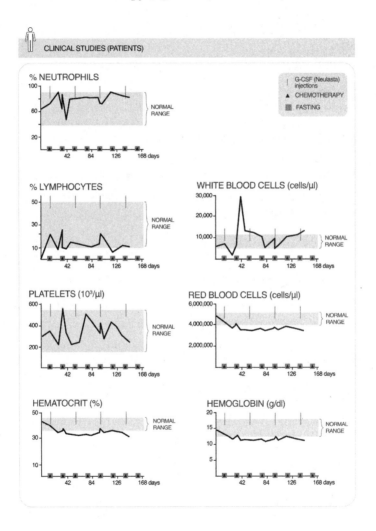

6.6. *The patient was able to maintain normal levels of (1) white blood cells, including neutrophils and lymphocytes, as well as (2) platelets, (3) hemoglobin, and (4) hematocrit. Maintaining these levels is important in helping each blood cell perform its functions and avoiding blood transfusions. Modified from Fernando M. Safdie et al., "Fasting and Cancer Treatment in Humans: A Case Series Report,"* **Aging** *1, no. 12 (2009): 988–1007.*

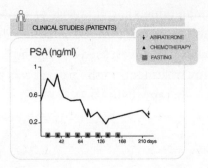

6.7. *The PSA level consistently decreased until the combined fasting and chemotherapy treatment was halted so the patient could be treated with hormone therapy (abiraterone). Modified from Fernando M. Safdie et al., "Fasting and Cancer Treatment in Humans: A Case Series Report,"* Aging *1, no. 12 (2009): 988–1007.*

These two case reports, along with the other studies described, indicate that fasting-mimicking diets can be combined with prostate cancer therapies, although clinical trials are necessary to determine whether a fasting-mimicking diet can reduce the side effects and increase the efficacy of standard prostate cancer therapies.

OTHER NUTRITIONAL THERAPIES IN PROSTATE CANCER TREATMENT

Obesity is a known risk factor for cancer, including prostate cancer, and it is associated with advanced stages of the disease. In men, just as we saw in the studies conducted on mice described earlier in the chapter, calorie restriction, in which patients were fed around five hundred to eight hundred calories per day, did not impact prostate cancer growth in overweight and obese men scheduled for radical prostatectomy (i.e., complete removal of the prostate).[8]

When protein-restricted diets were studied, there was evidence of their effect in reducing disease risk factors. In particular, patients with prostate cancer saw their insulin and leptin response improved and their PSA numbers lowered.[9]

Carbohydrate restriction also seems to positively affect PSA level in prostate cancer. A randomized, controlled trial involving six months of carbohydrate restriction examined overweight patients with prostate cancer and evaluated its impact on cancer recurrence. Out of a total of fifty-seven men, thirty-one were randomized to follow a low-carbohydrate diet (less than or equal to twenty grams per day) and twenty-six were assigned a control diet. While both groups consumed similar proteins and fats, those on the low-carbohydrate diet saw a reduction of weight (around 12 kilograms or 26.5 pounds in the low-carbohydrate group in six months versus 0.5 kilogram or 1 pound in the control diet group), HDL ("good" cholesterol), triglycerides, and HbA1c (glycated hemoglobin, which is a marker for the amount of blood sugar). Moreover, the number of months it would take for blood PSA to double was significantly higher in the lower-carbohydrate diet group than in the control group (twenty-eight versus thirteen months), providing initial evidence that severe carbohydrate restriction can slow prostate cancer growth.[10]

Because the everyday Longevity Diet is ideal in keeping blood sugar and amino acid levels low, but it is expected to be easier than the low-carbohydrate diet for most patients, it will be important to test its potential impact against prostate cancer cells compared with the low-carbohydrate diet.[11] Fasting and fasting-mimicking diets also have the potential to be effective in the management of prostate cancer, particularly in combination with cancer drugs targeting escape pathways. In conclusion, we have presented just a few case reports illustrating potential benefits, along with an interesting clinical study showing the feasibility of this approach in men with prostate cancer suffering from metabolic impairment caused by hormonal treatments.

PROSTATE CANCER TREATMENT SUMMARY

- Follow standard cancer therapy, which often involves hormone therapy but may employ many other types of therapy (chemotherapy, radiotherapy, surgery, etc.).
- Talk to your oncologist about combining a fasting-mimicking diet with the treatment plan.
- During treatment, follow the Longevity Diet (see chapter 3).
- Fast for thirteen to fourteen hours a day (by eating only, for example, between 8:00 a.m. and 6:00 p.m.) during therapy.
- Maintain a healthy body weight.
- Be physically active and exercise, after consulting your oncologist.
- Try to keep your phase angle (an indicator of muscle function) above 5 by doing muscle strength training for at least three or four times a week for thirty to forty minutes; you can follow the exercise video on the Create Cures website's section "Exercise and Longevity."

Patients who would like to learn more about the fasting/nutrition-based interventions described in this chapter should contact the Longevity and Healthspan Clinic of the Create Cures Foundation.

7

FASTING, NUTRITION, AND COLORECTAL CANCER

For their contributions to and review of this chapter, I thank Heinz-Josef Lenz, MD, professor of medicine and preventive medicine at USC's Keck School of Medicine, J. Terrence Lanni Chair in Gastrointestinal Cancer Research, and codirector of the Center for Cancer Drug Development and coleader of the Translational and Clinical Sciences Program at USC Norris Comprehensive Cancer Center and USC's Keck School of Medicine; Filippo de Braud, MD, full professor of medical oncology and director of the Graduate School in Medical Oncology at the University of Milan and director of the Department of Medical Oncology and Hematology at the Istituto Nazionale dei Tumori in Milan; Ana Luísa de Castro Baccarin, MD, medical oncologist and founder of Instituto Ana Baccarin—Oncologia e Qualidade de Vida in São Paulo; and Lizzia Raffaghello, PhD, research biologist at the Giannina Gaslini Institute in Genoa.

COLORECTAL CANCER: WHAT IT IS AND HOW IT IS TREATED

Colorectal cancer is the third-most-common and one of the most lethal cancers in the world, with 1.9 million cases diagnosed in 2020.[1] Colorectal cancer develops in either the colon or the rectum, which are parts of the large intestine and constitute the end part of the digestive system. The colon is a tube about 1.5 meters (5 feet) long. In most cases, colorectal cancers begin within polyps, which can grow on the inside of the colon or rectum. These polyps are often benign (adenomas) but can become cancerous over time.

Treatment strategies include chemotherapy (fluoropyrimidine, oxaliplatin, irinotecan, and trifluridine/tipiracil) and biologic agents (anti-VEGF: bevacizumab, aflibercept, ramucirumab, and rego-rafenib), which improve the overall survival rate.

Early-stage cancerous polyps can be surgically removed, while cancer that is stage II or higher is usually treated both surgically and with therapies that include chemotherapy, and in some cases in combination with radiotherapy. For stage IV colorectal cancer, in which the cancer has reached areas far from the colon or rectum (like the lungs), oncologists often recommend additional therapies that block specific targets that are very active in cancer, such as the vascular endothelial growth factor (VEGF), involved in the formation of the blood vessels that feed the cancer, or drugs like cetuximab or panitumumab that target other factors, like epidermal growth factor receptor (EGFR), a receptor involved in the growth of various types of cancer.

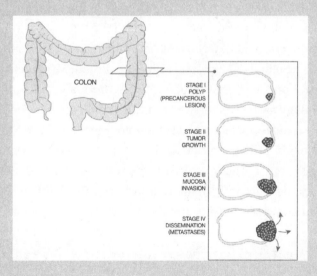

7.1. *Colorectal cancer is caused by the malignant transformation of polyps, which can be initially benign. In the various stages of the tumor, the polyp enlarges (stages II and III), spreading to the lymph nodes and subsequently also to other organs and creating metastases, especially in the liver and lungs (stage IV).*

. . . .

IN 1931, OTTO WARBURG, A biochemist and physician in Berlin, won the Nobel Prize in Physiology or Medicine in part for the discovery of what would later become known as the Warburg effect. It described the ability of cancer cells to become less dependent on the energy produced in the cell's mitochondria and to instead obtain energy by burning more sugars. It was not until much later that it was discovered that sugars are used rapidly by cancer cells not only to generate the "energy" to power the entire cellular activity but also to generate the key components of the cell, including DNA and other molecules that are needed for rapid cancer growth. So sugars provide both the energy and the carbons that become the "bricks" used to build new cells. Thus, it has been clear for a century that nutrients can affect cancer growth, but this general knowledge is not enough, and not surprisingly, its applications in the clinic have been minimal.

Although this is changing rapidly, nutrition has been historically viewed by many scientists and oncologists as an intervention of marginal or no importance, a lifestyle factor that may provide some help to the "real medicines" like chemotherapy, hormone therapy, or immunotherapy. One reason is that the goal of oncology trials is overall survival and progression-free survival, and it is very hard to perform robust trials to properly analyze the impact of nutritional interventions using standards that satisfy the FDA, which are best addressed by pharmacological drug interventions. For this reason, many of the oncologists who have helped me with this book have been testing a fasting-mimicking diet. In collaboration with some of the leading cancer hospitals around the world, we are now beginning to test the effect of fasting-mimicking-diet cycles on overall survival and progression-free survival, including in colorectal cancer in both animal and human studies.

. . . .

FASTING, FASTING-MIMICKING DIET, AND COLORECTAL CANCER TREATMENT

It's been a hundred years since the discovery of the importance of sugar for cancer cells, but it's only now that we are beginning to see interest in how nutrition—in particular, fasting and other dietary restrictions—affects whether cancer occurs and how we treat it. The reason it took so long is that reducing sugars alone does not hurt cancer cells enough or in many cases at all. Also, normal cells depend on sugar, and some normal cells, such as neurons, just like cancer cells, depend on high levels of sugars.

In 2012, together with graduate student Changhan Lee, we published a study combining the use of fasting and the chemotherapy drug doxorubicin to treat colorectal cancer cells in my laboratory in Los Angeles. However, the study didn't show any ability of fasting to make colon cancer cells more sensitive to this particular chemotherapy drug. While fasting alone can be as effective as chemotherapy against certain cancer types, including some colon cancer cells, we saw no effects.[2] It wasn't until years later that we demonstrated that fasting worked very well against colorectal cancer when it was used in combination with another chemotherapy drug, which is much more commonly used to treat colorectal cancer (oxaliplatin, see below).

Therefore, the fasting-mimicking diet needs to be applied based on the understanding of the specific molecular and metabolic functions of cancer cells, allowing it to be combined with the most effective drugs. It is also very important to consider the mechanism of action of each drug, because some perform better under fasting conditions. Over the last ten years, we have made significant progress in identifying biomarkers that predict the efficacy of targeted drugs and chemotherapeutic regimens. Oncology is moving toward increasingly personalized treatment strategies, using the ability to determine cancer's DNA sequence, the number of circulating cancer cells, or how cancer cells are rewired upon treatment. Understanding the molecular characteristics of each colon cancer cell is critical to developing the most personalized and effective intervention.

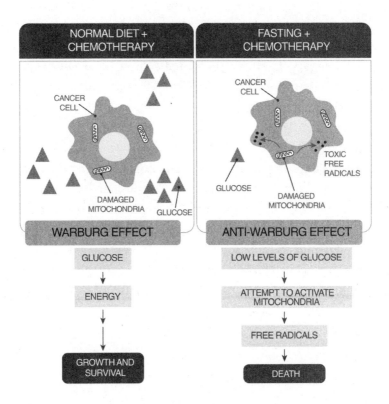

7.2. *The combustion engine of the cells, where energy is produced, the mitochondria, are damaged in most cancer cells. The Warburg effect is the attempt by cancer cells, which cannot rely on this engine, to produce energy and other molecules from nutrients and in particular from sugar without using mitochondria. During fasting, the cancer cell struggles to produce energy from the mitochondria but now is also not able to get a sufficient level of sugars, producing instead high levels of free-radical toxins, which cause the cancer cell to die. This anti–Warburg effect seems to be occurring in different types of cancer cells. Modified from Giovanna Bianchi et al., "Fasting Induces Anti-Warburg Effect That Increases Respiration but Reduces ATP-Synthesis to Promote Apoptosis in Colon Cancer Models,"* Oncotarget *6, no. 14 (2015): 11806–19.*

THE "ANTI-WARBURG EFFECT"

In our early experiments, when we starved cancer cells and treated them with chemotherapy, we observed a significant increase in "free radicals," toxic molecules that can damage DNA and many other components of the cell. Thanks to the work of graduate student Giovanna Bianchi and researcher Lizzia Raffaghello at the Gaslini children's hospital in Italy, we hypothesized that, by lowering blood sugars, fasting would force colon cancer cells to try to reverse the Warburg effect (cancer cells producing energy from sugar while reducing the need for mitochondria) in order to return to generating energy from the normal powerhouse of the cell: the mitochondria. In fact, fasting caused what we eventually named the "anti–Warburg effect": it pushed the cells to attempt to get more energy from the mitochondria. The problem is that this part of the cancer cell is severely damaged and, in most cases, no longer able to produce energy, or at least to produce a sufficient level of energy. We noticed that the fasted cancer cells made even less energy but instead produced high levels of free-radical toxins, which rapidly killed them. Thus, in a desperate attempt to survive, cancer cells commit suicide (figure 7.2).

FASTING, FASTING-MIMICKING DIET, AND NOVEL THERAPIES AGAINST COLORECTAL CANCER

Chemotherapy can kill cancer cells, but it can also kill many healthy cells, especially those that grow rapidly, such as hair cells or those on the inside of the gut. Researchers have been putting great effort into developing "smarter" drugs that target specific receptors or pathways tumors depend on. These types of drugs—for instance, antibodies that block the function of a particular cellular pathway—don't have the same level of side effects that chemotherapy drugs do. In addition to antibodies, researchers have developed small molecules, known as kinase inhibitors, that target activated

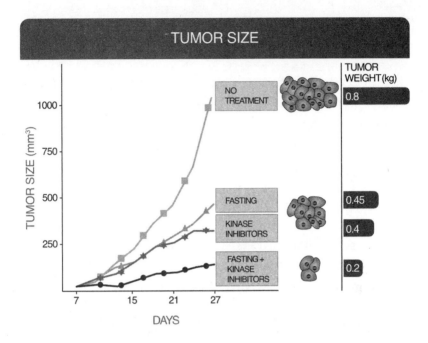

7.3. *Fasting boosts the activity of the kinase inhibitor, which targets activated growth genes in cancer cells of mice with colorectal cancer. Kinases are enzymes that activate growth signals. Modified from Irene Caffa et al., "Fasting Potentiates the Anticancer Activity of Tyrosine Kinase Inhibitors by Strengthening MAPK Signaling Inhibition," Oncotarget 6, no. 14 (May 20, 2015): 11820–32.*

growth pathways highly active in certain cancers. The great majority of cancer cells have constitutively active kinases—enzymes locked in "always on" mode, often because of DNA mutations. Kinase inhibitors block these high-traffic cancer highways and can be effective in either stopping the growth of cancer cells or even killing them.

In collaboration with the University of Genoa and the Gaslini children's hospital in Italy, my laboratory showed that fasting cycles made these kinase inhibitors more effective against colon cancer cells, indicating that fasting and the fasting-mimicking diet may be effective when combined with many cancer drugs other than chemotherapy (figure 7.3).[3]

NONTOXIC ANTIAGING THERAPIES
THAT ALSO KILL CANCER CELLS

Vitamin C was first made famous for its antiaging properties by chemist and winner of two Nobel Prizes (one for chemistry and one for peace) Linus Pauling, who was a professor at the California Institute of Technology in Pasadena, fifteen miles away from my university in Los Angeles. Pauling himself took several grams of vitamin C every day. Pauling was also among the first to suggest that vitamin C could be used to treat cancer. He knew that vitamin C can increase the production of the toxic free radicals. However, the weak results obtained in the clinic when only high doses of vitamin C were injected into cancer patients limited the interest in this vitamin until 2015, when the Lewis Cantley laboratory pub-

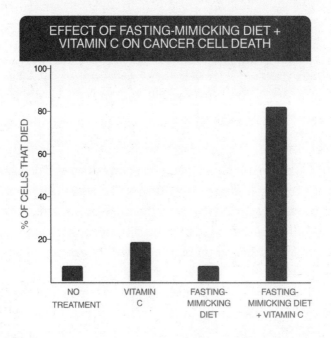

7.4. *In different types of colorectal cancer cells, vitamin C alone has a limited or moderate effect in killing cancer cells. However, vitamin C in combination with the fasting-mimicking diet has a much greater ability (up to ten times more) to kill cancer cells. Modified from Maira Di Tano et al., "Synergistic Effect of Fasting-Mimicking Diet and Vitamin C Against KRAS Mutated Cancers,"* Nature Communications 11, no. 1 (May 11, 2020): 2332.

lished a mouse study in *Science* magazine[4] describing how vitamin C was effective against colorectal cancer with specific mutations that activate the RAS pathway, one of the pathways that I discussed earlier.

In an attempt to generate a nontoxic anticancer intervention similar to antibiotics, we wanted to know whether the fasting-mimicking diet could make vitamin C more effective against cancer. Thanks to the funding from an AIRC (Italian Association for Cancer Research) grant, Maira Di Tano tested this with colorectal cancer as well as with a variety of cancers that had a KRAS mutation (KRAS is a gene that is reported to be present in nearly 30 percent of all cancers).[5] The study confirmed that vitamin C alone had a small to moderate effect in killing cancer cells, but when vitamin C was combined with the fasting-mimicking diet, its ability to kill cancer cells increased up to tenfold in three different types of human and mouse colorectal cancer cells (figure 7.4).[6]

Why was the combination of fasting and vitamin C so effective at killing cancer cells? Typically, when vitamin C and the iron within human cells encounter each other, they can generate toxic levels of oxygen free radicals that kill the cell (figure 7.5). But in my lab, Maira Di Tano discovered that cancer cells treated with vitamin C increased the production of ferritin, a factor that acts as a sponge for iron, preventing it from reacting with vitamin C and thus avoiding the generation of the free radicals that can kill the cells. Thus, vitamin C causes some toxicity to the cancer cells, but this toxicity is low because high levels of ferritin are produced. Fasting reduces the ferritin, therefore making the vitamin C very toxic but only to cancer and not normal cells.

However, combining vitamin C and fasting cycles was not enough to cure the mice, and it was only when Di Tano added chemotherapy that she started to see an even more powerful effect on cancer (figure 7.6).

Because fasting, together with vitamin C and chemotherapy, does not cure mice with colorectal cancer, my lab started to focus on identifying the escape pathways of colorectal cancer cells, as

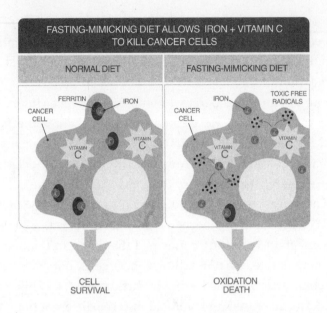

7.5. *Under normal feeding conditions, ferritin is bound to iron and prevents vitamin C from reacting with it. During fasting, ferritin decreases and free iron levels increase, allowing iron to react with vitamin C, generating toxic levels of free radicals that kill the cancer cell. Modified from Maira Di Tano et al., "Synergistic Effect of Fasting-Mimicking Diet and Vitamin C Against KRAS Mutated Cancers,"* Nature Communications *11, no. 1 (May 11, 2020): 2332.*

we had already done successfully for breast and other cancer types, so we can better identify a combination of nontoxic drugs that may provide remission in patients.

In 2020, M. L. Weng and collaborators confirmed that fasting and the fasting-mimicking diet can be combined with the kinase inhibitor rapamycin to achieve long-term survival in a mouse with colorectal cancer (figure 7.7). Notably, rapamycin is one of the predominant drugs able to extend life span in mice by inhibiting the mTOR-S6K signaling pathway, whose central role in aging was discovered by my laboratory in 2001.[7] However, in both mice and humans, rapamycin causes elevated blood glucose levels, which can promote cancer growth. Thus, the combination of the

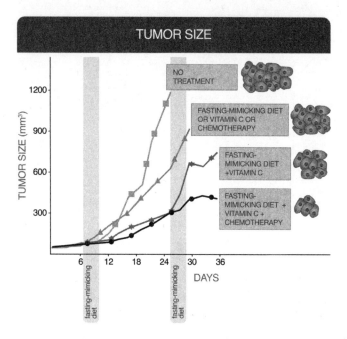

7.6. *Vitamin C combined with fasting-mimicking-diet cycles delays cancer growth in mice but is not enough to stop it. The two are more effective when combined with chemotherapy. Modified from Maira Di Tano et al., "Synergistic Effect of Fasting-Mimicking Diet and Vitamin C Against KRAS Mutated Cancers,"* Nature Communications *11, no. 1 (May 11, 2020): 2332.*

fasting-mimicking diet and rapamycin can increase the protection of normal cells against chemotherapy but also slow the growth of cancers that are stimulated either by mTOR-S6K activity or by high levels of sugars.

Like rapamycin, dexamethasone, which is widely used to reduce side effects in cancer patients, increases glucose levels. Therefore, it is worth discussing with an oncologist the potential use of the fasting-mimicking diet together with these drugs to lower blood glucose levels and possibly reduce side effects and delay cancer growth.[8]

. . . .

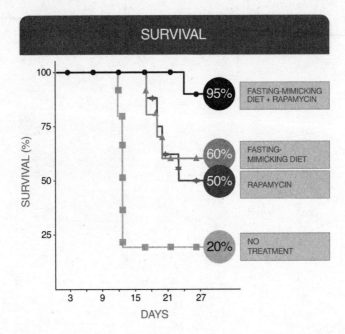

7.7. *Total survival rate of mice with colon cancer during normal diet and during fasting, with or without rapamycin. This is one of the main drugs that can extend the life span of mice by inhibiting the aging-accelerating pathway called mTOR-S6K. Modified from M. L. Weng et al.,* Nature Communications *11, no. 1 (2020): 1869.*

FASTING, FASTING-MIMICKING DIET, AND COLORECTAL CANCER: CLINICAL CASES

Unfortunately, we have not yet completed randomized clinical trials on the fasting-mimicking diet and colorectal cancer, but the potent effect in studies on mice, together with the promising preliminary clinical data, indicates that the fasting-mimicking diet has the potential to be an important enhancement of standard-of-care therapies.

In the ongoing trials, we did not see any significant side effects caused by the fasting-mimicking diet treatment with colorectal cancer patients. Colorectal cancer patients considering a fasting-mimicking diet in conjunction with therapy should discuss it with their oncologist first.

At the time of publication, there were two ongoing clinical trials investigating the effect of fasting on colorectal cancer. A Chinese group started a trial in 2020 in which 2,400 patients were recruited for a randomized study combining fasting with surgery to treat colorectal cancer.[9] The other trial, which also began in 2020, followed 100 patients with colorectal cancer in Madrid undergoing a short-term fasting period (forty-four to forty-eight hours), starting twenty-four hours before chemotherapy treatment.[10] Another trial carried out by Dr. Lenz and colleagues in collaboration with my group, combining vitamin C, the fasting-mimicking diet, and immunotherapy, will begin soon at USC.

In summary, the animal data for the use of fasting and the fasting-mimicking diet in combination with therapies ranging from chemotherapy to kinase inhibitors, as well as high-dose injected vitamin C, against colorectal cancer are very strong and have been confirmed by several laboratories. Also, some patients have been treated with this combination and have done very well, but clinical trials are ongoing and should be completed in the next few years.

Since the combination of vitamin C and the fasting-mimicking diet works best only for KRAS-mutated colorectal cancer cells, any patient should work with an experienced team before considering any dietary intervention.

Metastatic colorectal patients have high nutritional risk and sometimes a significant anabolic resistance, which means that caloric-restriction strategies could generate a catabolic process, worsening the disease prognosis. In the periods when they are off the fasting-mimicking diet cycles, patients should be closely monitored to guarantee adequate caloric and protein ingestion, as well as advised to perform resistance training regularly. Methods to measure and monitor muscle mass and strength should be taken into consideration. Chemotherapy also leads to many gastrointestinal side effects (nausea, vomiting, mucositis, diarrhea, and anorexia) that could aggravate the patient's nutritional risk.

· · · · · · ·

OTHER NUTRITIONAL THERAPIES IN COLORECTAL CANCER: THE GUT MICROBIOME IMPACT

The influence that certain dietary mediators, as well as chemical exposure and antibiotic consumption, exert over the intestinal microbiota (i.e., the microorganisms in the gut) and colorectal cancer risk is well known. Gut microbiota also have an important role in colorectal cancer development and progression.

For example, patients with colorectal cancer usually have an imbalance in gut bacteria, namely a deficit in beneficial bacteria but plenty of detrimental bacterial populations (proinflammatory pathogens). This imbalance can create subclinical (not detectable) and chronic inflammation that increases DNA mutation, thus promoting colorectal cancer growth.[11]

A personalized diet that modulates the gut microbiome pattern, such as one rich in high-fiber, polyunsaturated fatty acids, polyphenols, and probiotics (like a plant-pescatarian diet), may be a promising approach to increase the effectiveness of antitumoral therapy, as discussed in a review published in *Cancers* in May 2020.[12]

For example, a clinical trial with forty patients published in *Nature Communications* in 2015 concluded that a high-fiber diet promoted the diversification of gut flora and decreased the biomarker for cell proliferation and inflammation.[13]

A study of 992 stage III colon cancer patients following the American Cancer Society's Nutrition and Physical Activity Guidelines for Cancer Survivors (which consists of healthy body weight maintenance, physical activity, and a diet that includes vegetables, fruits, and whole grains) displayed a 42 percent lower risk of death during the study period and a higher five-year survival rate.[14]

Another literature review supports high-fiber diets in colon cancer patients on immunotherapy, providing the basis to further investigate in future research the role of dietary intervention in improving cancer outcomes.[15] Also, metagenomic analysis (the study of microbes directly in their environment) of stool by 16S rRNA gene sequencing is an evolving field of research and in the future will allow physicians to elaborate personalized therapeutic approaches to modulate each patient's gut microorganisms.[16]

More research is needed regarding the role of the fasting-mimicking diet and other nutritional interventions in colorectal cancer, but the available results are promising.

Following is a case report of an exceptional response from the clinical trial conducted by Francesca Ligorio and her collaborators,[17] as well as three patients' stories to show the importance of teamwork and having a combination of traditional and integrative (nutritional and lifestyle) treatments.

Case Report

In July 2016, a forty-seven-year-old man underwent a transverse colectomy for KRAS-mutated colorectal cancer. After eight cycles of capecitabine/oxaliplatin adjuvant chemotherapy, a PET (positron emission tomography) scan revealed disease relapse with metastases in the peritoneum.

The patient was then enrolled in a clinical trial on a fasting-mimicking diet and since August 2017 has received twelve cycles of first-line capecitabine-irinotecan (XELIRI) chemotherapy plus bevacizumab in combination with eight triweekly fasting-mimicking diet cycles, followed by maintenance therapy with capecitabine-bevacizumab for an additional six months. Two months after the initiation of the study treatment, a PET scan revealed a complete remission (no evidence of the cancer) (figure 7.8).

Despite treatment interruption in August 2018, complete tumor response was maintained until January 2021, when the PET scan revealed the recurrence of an active cancer. At that time, chemotherapy plus bevacizumab (which blocks the growth of blood vessels) in combination with cyclic fasting-mimicking diet was resumed. Notably, the treatment resulted in a new complete remission, which is still ongoing.

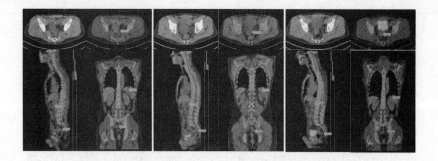

Week 186, PD
18-FDG PET scan

Week 42 (retreatment)
18-FDG PET scan

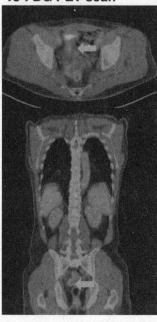
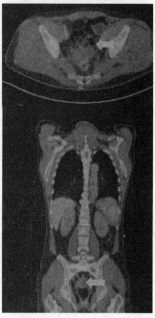

7.8. *A PET scan to detect tumor activity (arrows) in a patient treated with fasting-mimicking-diet cycles plus standard therapy at weeks 0 (baseline before therapy), and at different time points during treatment (weeks 14 and 146). Two months after the initiation of the study treatment, a PET scan revealed a complete remission (no evidence of the cancer) maintained for about three years, despite treatment interruption. After recurrence of the cancer (week 186), new cycles of the fasting-mimicking diet plus standard-of-care treatment were administered, showing a new complete remission (week 42), which was still ongoing at the time of writing this chapter. From Francesca Ligorio et al., "Exceptional Tumour Responses to Fasting-Mimicking Diet Combined with Standard Anticancer Therapies: A Sub-Analysis of the NCT03340935 Trial,"* European Journal of Cancer *172 (September 2022): 300–310.*

PATIENTS' STORIES AND EXPERIENCES

Clinical Case of Metastatic KRAS-Mutated Rectal Cancer

Dr. Ana Luísa de Castro Baccarin:

As an oncologist, I am challenged daily with the finitude of life. When we are unable to provide a longer life, we aim to provide more quality of life. I also try to think in a multidimensional way, and in my practice, I offer a unique combination of care options focused on integrating nutrition and metabolic health to the conventional treatment of my patients. That's how I got to know Dr. Valter Longo and his colleagues' research and the fasting-mimicking diet. I was surprised by a paper by Dr. Longo's group that showed mice with a strong antitumor activity after the association of high-dose ascorbate (vitamin C) and the fasting-mimicking diet against mutated KRAS colon cancer.

In 2020, one of my patients developed a mutated KRAS metastatic colon cancer. There weren't many treatment options available, and the disease continued to progress. At the same time, the patient was clinically fine and able to receive additional therapy. My patient, forty-eight years old, was diagnosed in 2017 with metastatic rectal cancer that spread to the thyroid and liver. She started first with chemotherapy (FOLFIRINOX), then switched to FOLFOX and then FOLFIRI and bevacizumab. However, in September 2020, the disease progressed to the liver and lungs.

Based on the absence of new therapeutic targets and the paper published by Dr. Longo and colleagues, I proposed a modified scheme of treatment as follows: fasting-mimicking diet (five days) + chemotherapy + bevacizumab (a blocker of blood vessel growth) + vitamin C day 1 to day 3. Cycles were repeated every three weeks. CEA (a special marker for colorectal cancer), which at baseline in September 2020 was 2,436, dropped to 1,798 in November 2020. Tumor marker CA 19-9 remained stable. Another cancer marker, the lactate dehydrogenase (LDH) measure, dropped from 1,322 to 841.

It is worth noting that since the disease progressed in September 2020, this was the first time tumor markers had been reduced, and there was also an improvement in liver-function markers. The scheme was relatively well tolerated, with the most relevant side effect being fatigue at the end of the five-day cycle, which is already expected because of the oxidative stress generated by this kind of protocol. The patient's muscle mass remained stable throughout the cycles performed. In the period between cycles, the patient was encouraged to perform resistance training and eat a more protein-rich diet, predominantly from vegetable protein sources. For better control of appetite during the five days of a fasting-mimicking diet, 0.6 milligrams of liraglutide, a diabetes drug that also suppresses hunger, was added. Apparently, this strategy did not compromise the effectiveness of the protocol. For four months, my patient showed no evidence of the disease, and she was able to spend another Christmas with her family.

Unfortunately, in January 2021, we noticed an increase in tumor markers and liver enzymes. New exams were performed, revealing disease progression in the liver and lungs. In December 2020, the combination of new cancer drugs trifluridine + tipiracil had been approved in Brazil and was thus given to the patient. In view of the progressive increase in tumor markers and clinical worsening, palliative care was proposed in April 2021.

Even though eventually the cancer came back, the patient was able to have another four months when no oncological guidelines said it would be possible. No single drug in the context of her disease would have achieved this gain and her case will certainly inspire other doctors and patients. The complexity of cancer shows that the future of oncology is the adoption of an equally complex approach, where several

tumor-activation pathways must be managed together.
Metabolic support for cancer therapy is a fascinating
therapeutic tool, and I am grateful to have benefited from Dr.
Longo's research.

REGARDING THE CASE ABOVE, I wonder what would have happened if, when the cancer came back, the patient had gone back to the vitamin C + fasting-mimicking-diet-based therapy. The colorectal cancer patient in the Ligorio study went into remission thanks to the use of a therapy that included the fasting-mimicking diet plus several drugs. Years later, the cancer returned, but he went back into another complete remission after using the same combination.

Gabriele, Switzerland

At age fifty-eight, Gabriele began to feel a lot of fatigue and was prescribed an iron injection, a gastroscopy, and a colonoscopy. A few days later, he received a phone call from his doctor, who gave him unexpected news: colon cancer. After further examinations (MRI and PET scan), three liver metastases were also discovered. He was shocked because he lived a healthy lifestyle: he maintained a normal weight, didn't smoke, rarely drank alcohol, and played sports.

Gabriele did some research and discovered many stories of people who fasted during chemotherapy. He opted for an interval of thirty-six hours before and thirty-six hours of fasting after the oxaliplatin infusion, only after their oncologist's approval. He changed his daily diet by eliminating certain dairy products and sugar.

From February through October, as he underwent chemotherapy and two surgeries, he followed this diet (with fasting) and experienced some classic adverse effects (headache, metallic taste, fatigue, diarrhea, etc.) during the first course of chemotherapy. But luckily, for the remainder of the therapy, he had no other adverse drug-related effects and was able to continue going on daily walks. After treatment, he regained weight and, after twenty physiotherapy sessions, resumed skiing and is working part time as a computer scientist.

Massimiliano Longo

Massimiliano is a renowned creative director who was diagnosed with stage IV colon cancer at the age of forty-three. After a complex surgery in which thirty-three centimeters of colon, part of the peritoneum (a membrane that covers the abdominal cavity), and sixty-five lymph nodes were removed, he came to the Valter Longo Foundation clinic in Milan, where Dr. Romina Inés Cervigni gave him recommendations on everyday nutrition. She also put him in contact with doctors who were conducting a clinical study at the San Martino Hospital in Genoa combining fasting-mimicking diet with standard therapy.

In just a few short months Massimiliano had implemented a multipronged strategy to deal with his cancer: standard care (surgery and twelve cycles of chemotherapy), the fasting-mimicking diet, various supplements to counteract the neurotoxic effects of the chemotherapy, genetic analysis, and pain therapy with medical cannabis. Between cycles of chemotherapy, he also followed the Longevity Diet.

This strategy helped him through his treatment. At the time of publication, Massimiliano was still undergoing additional chemotherapy cycles, but he was facing the moment as courageously as ever.

COLORECTAL CANCER TREATMENT SUMMARY

- Follow standard cancer therapy (surgery, chemotherapy, kinase inhibitors, etc.).
- Talk to your oncologist about combining therapy with a fasting-mimicking diet.

- Talk to your oncologist about following a high-dose injected vitamin C experimental therapy (if the cancer is KRAS mutated or similar).
- Between treatments, follow the Longevity Diet (see also chapter 3 about prevention).
- Fast for thirteen to fourteen hours a day (for example, eating only between 8:00 a.m. and 6:00 p.m.) during therapy, making sure to maintain normal muscle mass and healthy body weight.
- Be physically active and exercise, after consulting an oncologist.
- Try to keep your phase angle (an indicator of muscle function) above 5 by doing muscle strength training at least three or four times a week for thirty to forty minutes; you can follow the exercise video on the Create Cures website's section "Exercise and Longevity."

Patients who would like to learn more about the fasting/nutrition-based interventions described in this chapter should contact the Longevity and Healthspan Clinic of the Create Cures Foundation.

8

FASTING, NUTRITION, AND LUNG CANCER

For their contributions to and review of this chapter, I thank Filippo de Braud, MD, professor of medical oncology and director of the Graduate School in Medical Oncology at the University of Milan and director of the Department of Medical Oncology and Hematology at the Istituto Nazionale dei Tumori in Milan; Shadia Jalal, MD, associate professor of medicine at Indiana University; and Alessandro Laviano, MD, associate professor of medicine in the Department of Translational and Precision Medicine at Sapienza University of Rome.

LUNG CANCER: WHAT IT IS AND HOW IT IS TREATED

Lung cancer is the leading cause of cancer death in industrialized countries. In the United States, it is the most common cause of cancer deaths in men, and it has now surpassed breast cancer as the leading cause of death in women, according to the American Cancer Society.[1] Lung cancer incidence increases with age: the median age of patients is between sixty and seventy years at the time of diagnosis.

What are the main causes and risk factors for lung cancer?

1. Cigarette smoking. It is widely recognized that cigarette smoking is one of the main causes of lung cancer. Accord-

ing to the Centers for Disease Control and Prevention (CDC), smoking even a few cigarettes per day increases lung cancer risk, making it fifteen to thirty times higher.[2] Lung cancer risk drops five years after quitting smoking, yet it remains more than three times higher than the risk for those who have never smoked, even twenty-five years after quitting, according to a recent study published by the *Journal of the National Cancer Institute* with nearly nine thousand participants. Nonsmokers are also at risk from secondhand cigarette smoke.[3]

2. Exposure to radon. The International Agency for Research on Cancer (IARC) has classified radon, a radioactive chemical agent that contaminates indoor air worldwide, as an important risk factor that can increase cancer incidence in smokers. Radon's main source is the ground, from which it escapes and disperses into the environment, accumulating in closed rooms.

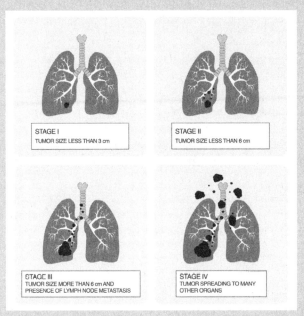

STAGE I
TUMOR SIZE LESS THAN 3 cm

STAGE II
TUMOR SIZE LESS THAN 6 cm

STAGE III
TUMOR SIZE MORE THAN 6 cm AND
PRESENCE OF LYMPH NODE METASTASIS

STAGE IV
TUMOR SPREADING TO MANY
OTHER ORGANS

8.1. *Lung cancer can develop anywhere in the lungs, giving rise to a mass that obstructs the proper flow of air. In stages I and II, lung tumors are small and are usually treated with minimally invasive surgical intervention. Stage III usually involves metastases to the lymph nodes of the chest, while stage IV involves spreading to both lungs and to distant organs.*

3. Atmospheric pollution and exposure to toxic agents of industrial origin.[4]

As reported by the Centers for Disease Control and Prevention, malignant lung tumors are divided into two main groups:

1. Small-cell lung cancer (SCLC) or microcitomas (smaller cancer cell size), which account for approximately 15 to 20 percent of cases

2. Non-small-cell lung cancer (NSCLC) or nonmicrocitomas (larger cancer cell size), which account for approximately 70 percent of cases

The majority of patients in whom the cancer hasn't spread to the lymph nodes (stages I and II) are treated with minimally invasive surgery. Stage II patients who qualify for therapy following surgery are normally treated with platinum-based chemotherapy, as it has been shown to improve overall survival.[5]

For stage IIIA, the presence of metastases in the lymph nodes usually results in the patient receiving chemotherapy or, in some cases, chemotherapy and radiotherapy preceding surgery for patients who qualify. The goal of treatment before surgery is to shrink the tumors and to tackle micrometastatic disease and improve outcomes. Stage IIIA non-small-cell lung cancer is more variable and treatment decisions should involve medical oncology, thoracic surgery, and radiation oncology. Stages IIIB–IV are typically inoperable. Patients with stage IIIB are evaluated for concurrent chemotherapy with radiation followed by immunotherapy. Patients with stage IV will receive systemic therapy, i.e., therapy reaching all parts of the body, but radiation can also be used to control the symptoms and reduce the suffering that the primary tumor or metastases can cause, thus improving the quality of life.

A FEW YEARS AFTER WE published our original work on fasting and cancer in 2008, I got a call from a friend of a famous cancer researcher at a leading research hospital. The researcher had been diagnosed with advanced-stage lung cancer, was not responding well to the therapy, and had little time left to live. I suggested he utilize a combination of fasting and chemotherapy to potentially make the treatment work better. He did so, and a year later, he was doing so well that he was able to return to work. The five-year survival for lung cancer is around 10 percent, and his expected survival was probably much shorter, considering he was not responding well to the initial chemotherapy cycles. So his surviving for eight years after diagnosis of such an aggressive lung cancer is very unusual, indicating that it was likely the fasting cycles that increased survival (as we will see from a more formal case report below).

Another benefit of combining a fasting-mimicking diet with other cancer therapies is its potential to reduce side effects, which can be very severe in some patients, even life-threatening. In most cases, oncologists or clinical studies have reported improvements in the therapeutic effects and/or reduction in side effects when combining cancer therapy with a fasting-mimicking diet, but until additional clinical trials are complete, we won't know the consequence of this combination. In the case of the cancer researcher with lung cancer, it was clear to all of us, including the oncologist at his own hospital, that time was of the essence and he could not wait for more conclusive research. When facing an aggressive cancer at an advanced stage, patients and oncologists should consider a fasting-mimicking diet in combination with the standard drug treatment.

FASTING, FASTING-MIMICKING DIET, AND LUNG CANCER: LABORATORY STUDIES

In our 2008 and 2011 mouse studies, we did not look at lung cancers. A few years later, a Swiss group published a paper on the use of fasting in combination with chemotherapy against two types of cancers that affect the lung: (1) human mesothelioma, a malignant tumor of the mesothelium (the thin layer of tissue that covers the lungs and the inner wall of the chest), and (2) lung cancer.[6]

Focusing not only on cancer growth but also on the cure rate of the mice, the article showed the following results:

1. For mesothelioma (a) none of the mice receiving either chemotherapy alone or fasting cycles alone were cured, but (b) nearly 60 percent of those receiving chemotherapy plus fasting cycles were cured (figure 8.2).

2. For mice with tumor cells derived from a lung cancer patient, (a) none of the mice receiving either chemotherapy or fasting cycles alone were cured, but (b) nearly 40 percent of those receiving chemotherapy plus fasting cycles were cured (figure 8.2).

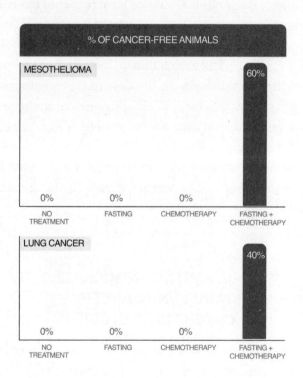

8.2. *Complete cancer remission in mice is observed only with a combined treatment of chemotherapy and fasting: (1) in 60 percent of animals with pleural mesothelioma, (2) in 40 percent of animals with lung adenocarcinoma cells (a subtype of non-small-cell lung cancer). Modified from Yandong Shi et al., "Starvation-Induced Activation of ATM/Chk2/P53 Signaling Sensitizes Cancer Cells to Cisplatin,"* BMC Cancer *12, no. 571 (2012).*

Once again, it was neither "starving" the cancer with fasting alone nor the standard treatment alone that worked best, but it was the combination of both, guided by the molecular understanding of how these treatments complement each other.

FASTING, THE FASTING-MIMICKING DIET, AND KINASE INHIBITORS

A few years later, in 2015, in collaboration with researchers at the University of Genoa, we showed that fasting was also very effective in making the kinase inhibitor crizotinib work more effectively against lung cancer cells. Specifically, crizotinib blocks certain growth signals in cells and consequently can block cancer cell growth. Because kinase-inhibitor drugs are part of a "targeted

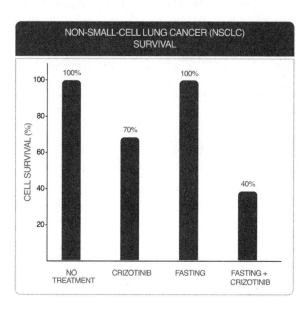

8.3. *The kinase-inhibitor drug crizotinib, combined with fasting, decreases survival of non-small-cell lung cancer (NSCLC) cells more effectively than crizotinib or fasting alone. Modified from Irene Caffa et al., "Fasting Potentiates the Anticancer Activity of Tyrosine Kinase Inhibitors by Strengthening MAPK Signaling Inhibition,"* Oncotarget 6, no. 14 *(2015): 11820–32.*

therapy"—a type of treatment that targets a very specific function in the cancer cell—this study confirmed that fasting and the fasting-mimicking diet could work with a wide variety of treatments, including targeted drugs in addition to the more toxic chemotherapy (figure 8.3).[7] However, even kinase inhibitors can be toxic, and as we have shown in our study on breast cancer led by Giulia Salvadori,[8] the fasting-mimicking diet was able to prevent their toxicity in mice (see chapter 4).

FASTING, FASTING-MIMICKING DIET, VITAMIN C, AND LUNG CANCER

The kinase inhibitors described above are less toxic than chemotherapy or radiotherapy, but they can still cause side effects. Also, they don't necessarily kill cancer cells but may simply block their growth as well as block the growth of normal cells. By exploiting our understanding of the differences between normal cells and cancer cells, we could use drugs that not only are nontoxic but could actually be protective for patients while being very toxic to cancer cells. As discussed in chapter 7, Maira Di Tano combined vitamin C with the fasting-mimicking diet, both of which are known to protect against aging and cellular damage, and applied them to lung cancer cells. Dr. Di Tano showed that this regimen was also very effective in killing different types of lung cancer cells (figure 8.4). Vitamin C or a fasting-mimicking diet alone caused a small increase in lung cancer cell death, but together they were very effective, killing lung cancer cells without damaging normal cells. Notably, this worked only if the cancer cells were of a specific but very common type: KRAS mutated.[9]

· · · · · · ·

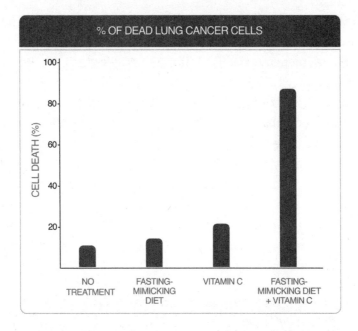

8.4. *Fasting and vitamin C together cause a major increase in the death of KRAS-mutated lung cancer cells. Modified from Maira Di Tano et al., "Synergistic Effect of Fasting-Mimicking Diet and Vitamin C Against KRAS Mutated Cancers,"* Nature Communications *11, no. 1 (2020): 2332.*

FASTING, FASTING-MIMICKING DIET, IMMUNOTHERAPY, AND LUNG CANCER

While immunotherapy—the use of drugs to stimulate the attack of cancer cells by the body's immune system—is one of the most promising cancer therapies today, most patients are not cured by it. Many also experience severe side effects, especially when multiple immunotherapy drugs are used. Laboratories are working on how to make immunotherapy more effective against cancer and applicable to more patients, and many strategies are beginning to show potential. Among them are fasting-mimicking-diet cycles, which we initially showed in 2016 to be effective in turning the immune system against breast cancer and melanoma, when combined with chemotherapy in mice,[10] a finding that is beginning to be confirmed in humans.[11]

One of the most effective immunotherapies involves the use of drugs that block PD-1, a protein found on a type of immune cells called T cells. PD-1 normally prevents the immune cells from attacking other cells. Immunotherapy removes this protection from cancer cells. One limitation of immunotherapy drugs is that they don't target only cancer cells and can affect both cancer and normal cells, thus providing an opportunity for immune cells to attack various types of normal cells.

But what happens when you combine fasting or a fasting-mimicking diet with immunotherapy? Could a fasting-mimicking diet make immunotherapy more toxic to cancer cells and less toxic

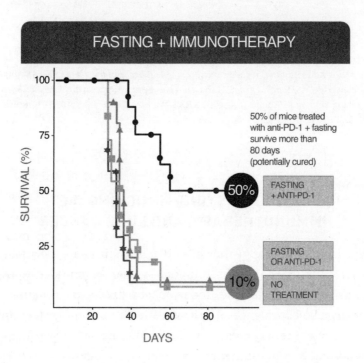

8.5. *Fasting in combination with immunotherapy (an anti-PD-1 drug) allows a survival of 50 percent of mice with lung cancer, without signs of cancer for at least eighty days. They are potentially cured. Modified from Daniel Ajona et al., "Short-Term Starvation Reduces IGF-1 Levels to Sensitize Lung Tumors to PD-1 Immune Checkpoint Blockade,"* Nature Cancer *1 (2020): 75–85.*

to normal cells? The first study to find out was done in 2020 by the laboratory of Rubén Pío Osés and colleagues at the University of Navarra in Spain; they combined fasting with an anti-PD-1 drug, one of the major immunotherapy drugs. The anti-PD-1 drug alone had not worked against lung cancers in mice.[12] The cancer grew at the same rate whether the immunotherapy was used or not. However, when mice fasted for several days in combination with immunotherapy, not only did the tumor not grow, but about 50 percent of the mice went into remission, without signs of cancer for at least eighty days (figure 8.5).

FASTING, FASTING-MIMICKING DIET, AND LUNG CANCER: CLINICAL STUDIES AND REPORTS

In our initial 2009 clinical report on fasting and cancer, one of the ten patients we followed had been diagnosed with a poorly differentiated non-small-cell lung carcinoma stage IV lung cancer,[13] which had spread to the bones, liver, spleen, and pancreas.

The patient was given the chemotherapy drugs docetaxel + carboplatin every twenty-one days. She was on a regular diet during the first five chemotherapy cycles and lost approximately four pounds each cycle. She reported returning to her normal weight within three weeks. Other side effects included severe muscle spasms, fatigue, numbness, easy bruising, and bowel discomfort. During the sixth cycle the patient fasted for forty-eight hours before and twenty-four hours after chemotherapy. She lost approximately six pounds during the fasting period, but this time recovered the weight within ten days. Unlike with previous cycles, after this cycle, the patient complained only of mild fatigue and weakness.

The side effects reported by the patient were reported to be consistently reduced when chemotherapy was administered together with a seventy-two-hour fasting period (figure 8.6). In the cycle in which she fasted, the patient reported that her strength returned more quickly than in previous cycles and that she was able to walk three miles only three days after the chemo cycle. The last scan, six months after the end of the chemo cycles, showed stable disease in the main mass in the lung and decreased disease activity in the spleen and liver compared with before the chemo cycles were started.

This case—together with the cases of lung cancer in the trials

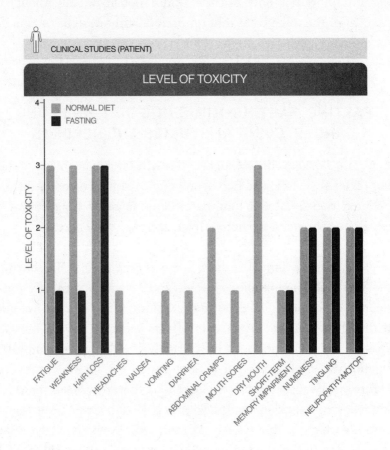

8.6. *The side effects of chemotherapy in a patient with stage IV lung cancer were reported to be stronger during the first cycles of chemotherapy, when the patient did not fast (gray bars), than during subsequent cycles, when she fasted in combination with chemotherapy (black bars). In some cases, side effects were absent when the patient fasted (for example, vomiting, diarrhea, mouth sores, headaches). Toxicity levels range from 0 (no toxicity) to 4 (high toxicity). Modified from Fernando M. Safdie et al., "Fasting and Cancer Treatment in Humans: A Case Series Report," Aging 1, no. 12 (2009): 988–1007.*

conducted by Claudio Vernieri and his collaborators[14] and Francesca Valdemarin and her collaborators,[15] in which patients were treated with both fasting-mimicking-diet cycles and a variety of therapies—indicate that fasting-mimicking-diet cycles combined with standard-of-care therapy are generally safe and potentially effective.

A Sixty-One-Year-Old Man with Extensive-Stage Small-Cell Lung Cancer[16]

After four cycles of chemotherapy, this patient was enrolled in the clinical trial to receive immunotherapy plus a cyclic fasting-mimicking diet. He completed eight triweekly cycles of this treatment without severe adverse events. He went into remission of pleural effusion (i.e., an accumulation of fluids between the layers of the pleura, tissue that lines the lungs and chest cavity) and lung and lymph node metastases, which was still ongoing forty months after the start of the treatment. Specific tumor biomarkers also became negative after three treatment cycles, and thereafter they remained within the normal range (figure 8.7).

Other studies have focused on the role of blood glucose levels on cancer progression. Juhua Luo and her collaborators studied 342 patients with non-small-cell lung cancer (NSCLC) and reported that those with fasting glucose levels above 126 mg/dl had a 69 percent increased risk of death compared with those who had normal glucose levels (below 99 mg/dl).[17] Although this study was not on the effect of fasting and the fasting-mimicking diet on lung cancer progression, we know from multiple human clinical trials that fasting-mimicking-diet cycles can reduce glucose and in many pre-diabetic and diabetic patients lower it sufficiently to return to normal levels. The results above suggest that fasting cycles could affect mortality in lung cancer patients in part by reducing glucose levels, without considering other effects. Naturally, we would be able to confirm this only after large, randomized clinical trials.

Whereas fasting / fasting-mimicking-diet cycles are consistently seen to make things worse for cancer cells, low glucose is not

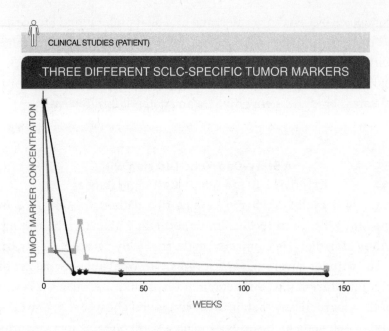

8.7. *Three tumor biomarkers decreased rapidly after starting the fasting-mimicking diet + immunotherapy cycles. Modified from Francesca Ligorio et al., "Exceptional Tumour Responses to Fasting-Mimicking Diet Combined with Standard Anticancer Therapies: A Sub-Analysis of the NCT03340935 Trial,"* European Journal of Cancer *172 (2022): 300–310.*

always found to be associated with a benefit for patients. Jin-Rong Yang and collaborators conducted a study in 2019 showing that patients with non-small-cell lung cancer who had blood glucose levels lower than 91 mg/dl displayed an increased risk of death compared with patients whose glucose was higher.[18] It is possible that this finding may be explained by frailty and possibly negative effects on immunity in patients with blood glucose levels lower than 91 mg/dl, possibly including those who are malnourished. This is another example of how cancer treatment and also the patient's health, independent of the cancer, are complex and are best handled by a team of experts. Notably, our collaborator and contributor to this chapter, oncologist Shadia Jalal at Indiana University, started a clinical trial in 2023 combining chemotherapy, immunotherapy, and the fasting-mimicking diet for the treatment of non-small-cell lung cancer.[19]

OTHER NUTRITIONAL THERAPIES IN LUNG CANCER: KETOGENIC DIET AND SUPPLEMENTS

We have discussed how ketogenic diets have been studied in combination with standard cancer therapy, especially for brain tumors, in both animal and human models. When it comes to lung cancer, though, studies have shown poor tolerance in patients with locally advanced non-small-cell lung carcinoma (NSCLC).

Researchers from the University of Iowa opened a phase I clinical trial in 2017 to assess the tolerability of a ketogenic diet combined with radiation and chemotherapy for approximately six weeks in inoperable patients with stage III and IV non-small-cell lung cancer.[20]

The ketogenic diet provided 90 percent of calories from fat, 8 percent from protein, and 2 percent from carbohydrates. Seven patients were enrolled in the study: two completed the clinical trial, four discontinued the ketogenic diet during therapy because of constipation, fatigue, bloating, and nausea, and one experienced a serious complication (abnormal levels of uric acid in the blood) and was removed from the study.

The low rate of completion indicates this particularly high-fat ketogenic diet is very difficult to complete in part because it causes a range of side effects, but this does not rule out the possibility of considering less extreme versions of ketogenic diets and of alternating them with a fasting-mimicking diet. When the patient needs more than standard therapies to treat very aggressive cancer types, such as lung cancer, oncologists and nutritionists may want to consider alternating between the Longevity Diet, a less extreme ketogenic diet, and the fasting-mimicking-diet cycles, with the goal to kill cancer cells while also minimizing muscle loss and frailty.

Several promising trials have also looked at the potential effects on lung cancer of supplementation with vitamins and essential fatty acids. In 2014, a randomized study was conducted in

Mexico focusing on nutritional, clinical, and inflammatory parameters, as well as quality of life, in advanced non-small-cell lung cancer patients receiving chemotherapy. Researchers compared two similar diets. The only difference was that one included an oral EPA (an enriched omega-3 fatty acid supplement) and the other did not. Ninety-two participants with non-small-cell lung cancer, aged between eighteen and eighty years, were included, some at stage IIIB (where cancer had spread to lymph nodes above the collarbone or to some nodes on the opposite side of the chest) and some at stage IV (where cancer had spread to the other lung or to other areas of the body). Patients were divided into two groups. Compared with the group who didn't take the EPA, patients receiving the supplement showed improved appetite and decreased fatigue and neuropathy, which is a dysfunction of one or more nerves resulting in pain, muscle weakness, numbness, or tingling in the affected area. Finally, results showed that the administration of an EPA could improve a general set of criteria that measure quality of life.[21] However, it is important to observe that there was no difference in response rate or overall survival between the groups.

Higher vitamin D levels are also associated with better survival in early-stage non-small-cell lung cancer. Nevertheless, because of the observational nature of this study, it is not possible to know if vitamin D levels affect survival in cancer patients or whether, for example, those who are healthier and responding better to therapies simply have higher vitamin D levels.

However, in a randomized, double-blind trial performed in Japan in 2018, which addressed the problem described above, 155 patients with non-small-cell lung cancer were randomly assigned to receive either vitamin D (1,200 IU per day) or a placebo, more for psychological than for physiological effects, for one year after surgery. Patients were then followed for approximately three years to understand whether this supplementation would improve their survival.[22] When they restricted the analysis to the subgroup with early-stage adenocarcinoma (cancer that begins in glandular secretory cells) with low 25(OH)D (25-hydroxyvitamin D), the vitamin D group showed significantly better five-year relapse-free survival (86 percent versus 50 percent) and overall survival (91 percent versus 48 percent) than the placebo group.

In general, specific supplements may be helpful for patients. However, unlike the cycles of fasting / fasting-mimicking diet, vitamins and other supplements have low potential to result in long-term remission, in part because they are not expected to greatly increase the death of cancer cells.

A PATIENT'S STORY AND EXPERIENCE

Maggie Jones

This patient wrote to me and eventually interviewed me as part of a documentary that focused on fasting and nutrition for cancer patients called *CANCER/EVOLUTION*. Here's her initial letter:

My name is Maggie Jones and I moved from Los Angeles to Hong Kong to start a new job one week before my 40th birthday. Exactly one month later, in October 2018, I was diagnosed with Stage IVB non-small-cell lung cancer that had metastasized to my brain and eye along with multiple lymph nodes throughout my chest and neck. This was quickly followed by more tumors in my brain, liver, and abdomen. At the time, the average life expectancy with treatment was 6–8 months and the 5-year survival rate was less than 1%. That is, it rounded to zero.

I grieved. For a couple of days, anyway. Then I started researching and decided that such a dire outcome didn't really apply to me. People do survive. One thousand is a little more than 0% of one million. I just needed to take control of what I could control, I thought.

So, I fasted for 24 hours during the weekend after my diagnosis and, when I resumed eating, I adopted a plant-based ketogenic diet, built around organic healing raw vegetables and oil.

After stumbling on some of the research by Professor Valter Longo on fasting, I started incorporating an 80 hour plus water fast each month.

After my first brain radiosurgery for two brain tumors in November 2018, I had a lot of weakness, shakiness, sweating, and vomiting for three weeks. So, before my second brain radiosurgery for two different tumors in April 2019, I did a water fast for three days. I was back at work within a few days after the procedure.

It has been six years since that diagnosis and four years and a

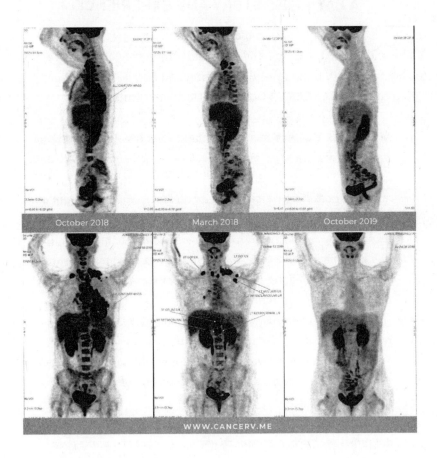

8.8. Computed tomography scans of Maggie from October 2018 to October 2019, showing the disappearance of cancer masses.

half since I received the news that there was "No Evidence of Disease." I am thrilled to be cancer free, but I did suffer some brain damage because of my treatments. Fasting was a vital tool for me to manage the adverse effects of my many medications and swelling, necrotic brain.

I now run cancerV.me, a company dedicated to spreading awareness of these lifesaving metabolic therapies and how to implement them. My upcoming documentary, entitled CANCER/ EVOLUTION, *promotes Professor Longo's research on nutrition and cancer because the principles he advocates are among those that I credit with my life.*

LUNG CANCER TREATMENT SUMMARY

- Follow standard cancer therapy (chemotherapy, radio-therapy, immunotherapy, targeted therapy, etc.).
- Talk to your oncologist about combining therapy with the fasting-mimicking diet.
- Between treatments, follow the Longevity Diet (see chapter 3). If this is not enough, talk with an oncologist and a nutritionist about combining the fasting-mimicking diet and the Longevity Diet with a plant-and-fish-based keto-genic diet, making sure that it won't adversely affect muscle mass or immune function.
- Talk to the oncologist about considering supplementation with vitamin D and omega-3 fatty acids. See also appendix 1.
- Fast for thirteen to fourteen hours a day (for example, eating only between 8:00 a.m. and 6:00 p.m.) during therapy.
- Maintain a normal body weight.
- Be physically active and exercise, after consulting with an oncologist.
- Try to keep your phase angle (an indicator of muscle function) above 5 by doing muscle strength training at least

three or four times a week for thirty to forty minutes; you can follow the exercise video on the Create Cures website's section "Exercise and Longevity."

Patients who would like to learn more about the fasting/nutrition-based interventions described in this chapter should contact the Longevity and Healthspan Clinic of the Create Cures Foundation.

9

FASTING, NUTRITION, AND BLOOD CANCERS

For his contributions to and revision of this chapter I want to thank Alessandro Laviano, MD, associate professor of medicine in the Department of Translational and Precision Medicine at Sapienza University of Rome.

BLOOD CANCERS: WHAT THEY ARE AND HOW THEY ARE TREATED

Blood cancers are commonly the result of mutations during the production of blood cells.[1] More than one million blood cancer cases occur every year worldwide, which can affect both children and adults. Common forms of blood cancers include the following:[2]

1. **Leukemia**, a cancer that starts in the blood-forming tissue, like bone marrow, and enters the bloodstream.

2. **Lymphoma**, a cancer deriving from the lymphocytes of the immune system.

3. **Myeloma**, a cancer deriving from the white blood cells that produce antibodies. Since antibodies are proteins produced by the immune system to protect the body from foreign substances (such as viruses, insect venoms, or

toxic materials), this cancer can alter the system's normal function.

These are just a few of the blood cancers; there are more than sixty distinct disease types, each having peculiar clinical features, treatment pathways, and outcomes.

The choice of the primary treatment to be used to fight a blood cancer depends on many factors, such as the specific characteristics of the tumor, the patient's age, and the general health of the patient, etc.

Chemotherapy remains the primary treatment, as well as radiotherapy, administered before a bone marrow transplant. Because chemotherapy and radiotherapy kill both leukemia cells and normal cells of the bone marrow, the transplant gives the patient either their own healthy stem cells or cells from a compatible donor. Immunotherapy has also been used to a lesser extent, and some targeted drug treatments have been developed to focus on blocking specific abnormalities present within cancer cells.

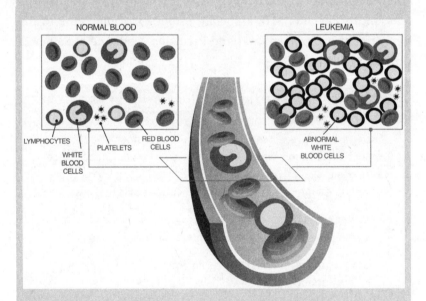

9.1. *Many blood cancers originate in the bone marrow, where blood cells (red blood cells, platelets, and white blood cells) are formed in part to fight infections. When blood cells accumulate specific DNA mutations, they can generate clones that cause a blood cancer, also disrupting their normal function.*

· · · · · · ·

IN 2012, I RECEIVED AN email from Woody Wright, who was working at University of Texas Southwestern Medical Center. A Harvard- and Stanford-trained MD and PhD, he had become famous in the aging field for pioneering studies on the role of telomeres (the end portions of chromosomes) and the Hayflick limit, which is the limit of human cells' ability to divide to generate identical cells.

In that email, he revealed that he had been diagnosed with multiple myeloma six years earlier, when one of the cervical vertebrae in his neck collapsed. He was treated with radiation and then with lenalidomide (Revlimid), a medication that reduces blood flow to kill the cancer cells. This treatment worked for more than

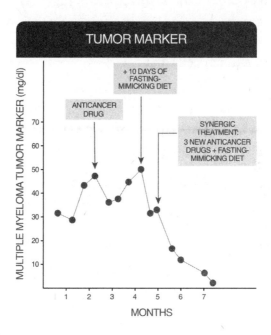

9.2. *Tumor marker levels show cancer progression in a patient suffering from multiple myeloma. After administration of the cocktail of drugs, the patient's cancer cells responded strongly. Despite this, the cancer became drug-resistant, and markers grew again. However, when the patient was placed on a ten-day fasting-mimicking diet plus the drugs, there was a remarkable response, indicating that cancer cells were sensitive to the combination of drugs with the fasting diet. Modified from an unpublished paper.*

three years, but then his cancer cells became resistant. The oncologist recommended a cocktail of drugs, which worked for a few months, but eventually the cancer became resistant to them, too. Woody, his oncologist, and I eventually wrote a case report (which we never submitted for publication) that pointed out that using "monotherapy"—a single or even a few drugs for the treatment of any cancer—will in most cases result in the "development of resistance." In January 2012, his oncologist gave him another cocktail of three drugs and his cancer cells responded dramatically, with his tumor marker going from 170 to less than 10. However, even with this triple treatment the cancer became resistant, and his numbers started to rise in May 2012. Woody then started cycles of the fasting-mimicking diet, first for five days and then eventually for ten days, in combination with several drugs. Even though the drugs he was taking were no longer effective on their own, following ten days of a fasting-mimicking diet created another dramatic response in the tumor cells (figure 9.2).

FASTING AND BLOOD CANCERS: LABORATORY STUDIES

Motivated in part by the cancer that was affecting Woody Wright, we published a study in 2015[3] that included both mice and clinical human data on the effects of cycles of the fasting-mimicking diet on longevity, disease, and/or risk factors for diseases. We treated mice starting at middle age (sixteen months old) with two cycles of a four-day-long fasting-mimicking diet per month until very old age (twenty-nine months old). In addition to extending the life span of the mice, the fasting-mimicking-diet cycles cut the incidence of tumors nearly in half and, importantly for purposes of this chapter, it reduced the incidence of one of the most common blood cancers: lymphoma. This cancer is particularly common in mice used in laboratory studies, and in our case, nearly 70 percent of mice on a normal diet developed a lymphoma during their life. In contrast, fewer than 40 percent of mice receiving fasting-mimicking-diet cycles for four days twice a month starting at middle age developed lymphomas (figure 9.3). We can conclude that fasting-mimicking-diet cycles alone had a major effect, but it isn't clear whether that was because they prevented lymphomas from forming or because they killed lymphoma cells after they were formed—perhaps both.

We had examined how fasting and fasting-mimicking-diet cycles alone could kill many different types of cancer cells in mice before, but we had not shown that they were effective in treating blood cancers. Maybe it was not surprising that, in 2017, laboratories at the same University of Texas Southwestern Medical

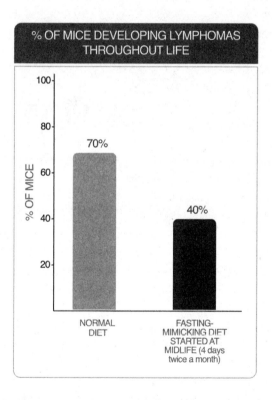

9.3. *Lymphoma incidence: lymphomas were formed in 70 percent of control mice but in only 40 percent of the fasting-mimicking-diet mice. Modified from Sebastian Brandhorst et al., "A Periodic Diet That Mimics Fasting Promotes Multi-System Regeneration, Enhanced Cognitive Performance, and Healthspan," Cell Metabolism 22, no. 1 (2015): 86–99.*

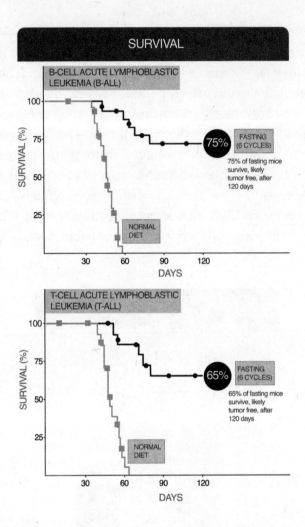

9.4. *Mice with acute lymphoblastic leukemia that affects B lymphocytes, white blood cells that usually fight infections (B-ALL), or T lymphocytes, white blood cells responsible for adaptive immune response (T-ALL), become apparently free of cancer when they fast. Modified from Zhigang Lu et al., "Fasting Selectively Blocks Development of Acute Lymphoblastic Leukemia via Leptin-Receptor Upregulation,"* Nature Medicine *23, no. 1 (January 2017): 79–90.*

Center Hospital, where Woody was a professor, published on the effects of fasting on blood cancers, in this case B and T cell acute lymphoblastic leukemia (B and T lymphocytes are cells of the immune system). They showed that fasting cycles alone inhibited leukemias from being formed, in agreement with our results, and reversed the progression of both B cell and T cell acute lympho-blastic leukemia (figure 9.4).[4]

However, fasting cycles alone did not work at all against acute myeloid leukemia (AML) (figure 9.5).[5]

Because fasting cycles alone could not prevent the deaths of more than a quarter of the mice, and considering their inefficacy against acute myeloid leukemia, these results are consistent with our proposal that fasting-mimicking-diet cycles should in most cases be combined with drugs to make the therapy more effective and also to block cancer cells from becoming resistant to fasting / fasting-mimicking diet alone. However, it cannot be ruled out that for some patients the fasting-mimicking diet on its own could be

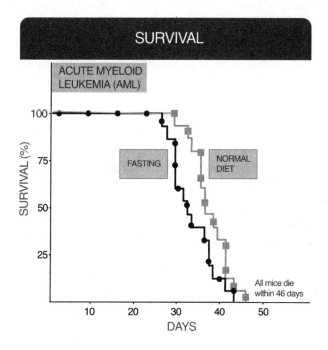

9.5. *Fasting cycles alone have no effect on the survival of mice with acute myeloid leukemia (AML). Modified from Zhigang Lu et al., "Fasting Selectively Blocks Development of Acute Lymphoblastic Leukemia via Leptin-Receptor Upregulation,"* Nature Medicine *23, no. 1 (January 2017): 79–90.*

useful, especially in the very early stages when chemotherapy or other treatments are not yet necessary.

FASTING AND BLOOD CANCERS:
CLINICAL CASES AND STUDIES

In a variety of cancers, animal studies have shown that treatments including fasting or the fasting-mimicking diet in tandem with drug therapy had potent anticancer effects. Furthermore, there have been several additional cases at other clinics that provide initial support for our studies on multiple myeloma, which showed fasting alone can be very effective against certain—but not all—blood cancers.

One study followed a forty-two-year-old woman diagnosed with grade 1 follicular lymphoma (stage IIIa, advanced stage) for three years. This is a slow-growing cancer of the lymphatic system that develops when the body makes abnormal B cells in the lymph nodes or other organs.[6] Her only treatment was a water-only fast for twenty-one days and then a plant-based diet free of refined carbohydrates and added salt, oil, and sugar. She did not receive any other cancer therapy. In the following years, CT and PET scans showed no signs of the cancer. The authors of the study report that the initial regression of the tumor coincided with the first water-only fast, suggesting, as indicated by the animal studies, that fasting may have been sufficient to treat this lymphoma.[7]

A word of caution: cancer patients should not take these findings as proof that fasting alone can cure cancer. I remember being very concerned after watching a documentary called *The Food Cure* in which I was interviewed, because in at least one and possibly several cases, cancer patients' conditions got worse or they died while refusing standard treatment and trying to cure cancer with food alone. Although fasting or extreme diets could cure or be effective against cancer in some cases, as we described above, both mouse and human studies indicate that combining fasting-mimicking diets with standard protocols is much more effective than either alone. Thus, to turn down such treatment in favor of fasting only can be very risky and is not advised.

However, in some cases when no standard-of-care treatment is recommended, dietary interventions may be an appropriate option. We have had several patients who have adopted the Longevity Diet, a periodic fasting-mimicking diet, or both against leukemia in the pretreatment "watch and wait" stage (when oncologists do not believe it is yet necessary to prescribe drugs). After years of following the fasting/dietary strategies, the patients did well and, at the time of this publication, have not needed chemotherapy or other drugs. While these results are very promising, they are very far from conclusive. We and others plan to perform clinical trials that will, we hope, confirm that fasting-mimicking diets and other nutrition-based interventions alone are effective in preventing the onset and possibly the progression of certain blood cancers in humans, as we have shown in mice. For cancer at stages for which fasting alone is not expected to be effective, a combination of the fasting-mimicking diet and specific drugs may be more effective in curing or keeping the cancer under control.

In addition to fasting, other nutritional therapies described below have been tested against blood cancers.

OTHER NUTRITIONAL
THERAPIES FOR BLOOD CANCERS

Diet has been shown to improve patients' quality of life, as reported in a study conducted on eighty-four patients.[8] They were divided into two groups: one received only antileukemic treatment, and the other antileukemic treatment and supplementation with antioxidants. Infectious complications were less frequent in the antioxidant group, possibly because of their effect in stimulating the immune system.

Another study, conducted on a cohort of 568 women with

non-Hodgkin's lymphoma (NHL), a cancer that starts in white blood cells, raises the possibility that eating more green leafy vegetables and citrus fruits could be useful in improving prognosis and survival, even if their effect on the course of the disease and survival appears to apply to only a portion of non-Hodgkin's lymphoma subtypes.[9]

We also have some anecdotal evidence that this can be a key strategy for patients who have decided, together with their oncologist, to combine a fasting-mimicking diet with their standard therapy.

PATIENTS' STORIES AND EXPERIENCES

Chris

Chris was diagnosed with chronic lymphocytic leukemia (CLL) in December 2009, with a slow but constant increase in her white blood cells (WBC) and her absolute lymphocyte count (ALC), two of the most important disease markers in CLL patients.

After reading an article about my research in Canada's *National Post*, Chris decided to experiment with a four-day water-only fast. Her cancer marker levels decreased, which had not happened before. She did four additional water-only fasts during the following year, prior to discovering the fasting-mimicking diet. She started the fasting-mimicking diet in 2017 and completed around five cycles every year. She watched her white blood cell and absolute lymph node numbers decrease to 2011 levels, and now she is in a stage of "watch and wait."

"Bottom line, at this point my blood counts are about where they were back in 2011. I asked my hematologist's nurse about this, and she informed me that they had not heard of such reversals with those following standard treatment," Chris said.

. . . .

"C."

After eighteen months and fifteen specialists, C. was diagnosed with polycythemia vera—a rare blood cancer in the bone marrow that causes increased production of red blood cells—in October 2012. In her case, there was also a common mutation in the JAK2 gene of this tumor.

In September 2017 she needed to start chemotherapy— Onco-Carbide tablets (at first, once a day for five days, then twice a day, six days a week). Side effects included gastrointestinal problems, fatigue, repeated vomiting and diarrhea, and extreme exhaustion. Her condition worsened, and she started to have fainting spells and was losing weight. "I used to describe these days of total blackout as if I had been hit by a car. The sensation of generalized pain throughout the body lasted for forty-eight hours," she reported.

At that time, a friend sent her a screenshot of a page from *The Longevity Diet*. It was a passage where I discussed the use of the fasting-mimicking diet against cancer. She tried it once, and afterward she decided to contact my foundation in Milan, where she participated in the clinical study of the Ospedale Policlinico San Martino in Genoa in November 2018.

C. followed the fasting-mimicking diet during chemotherapy. Several side effects disappeared, and she also saw a reduction of other adverse effects, including early onset of menopause.

"The pain of menopause associated with my condition could make my life hell," she said. "I had this cyclical opportunity to be reborn during the week of the fasting-mimicking diet."

"A.P."

In 2014 A.P. was a fit and healthy forty-six-year-old, a married and working mom of three. Suddenly, she started experiencing fatigue and dizziness—sometimes so severe that she would need to lie down and stay home from work. When she talked to her doctors, they first suspected she might have low iron. However, she soon experienced new symptoms like stomach swelling. After an investigation, she was diagnosed with stage IV non-Hodgkin's follicular lymphoma.

After a few days, she began her chemo (R-CVP, a combination of cancer drugs: rituximab, cyclophosphamide, vincristine, and prednisolone, a steroid). The first chemo treatment was not very successful in reducing tumor size, so her doctors decided she should have a more aggressive chemo course (R-CHOP, made up of rituximab, cyclophosphamide, hydroxydaunorubicin, vincristine, and prednisone), as well as a transplant of her own stem cells, and then radiotherapy.

It was at this stage that her husband stumbled across an article about my research in a UK newspaper. A.P. wrote to me in July 2015, and I gave her recommendations for her oncologist. Her oncologist was worried and refused to endorse fasting, so A.P. decided to change both hospital and oncologist. Her new, more experienced oncologist told her that, if she wanted to fast, she could manage it, and that he was more than happy and available to support her.

A.P. fasted for three days prior to treatment and one day following treatment. She was careful to go back to eating a regular diet after fasting so her weight would return to normal. Even though her R-CHOP therapy in combination with fasting was very aggressive and gave her the classic adverse effects of chemotherapy (hair loss, weakness, nausea), she tolerated the treatment well and did not feel any worse than she had during her first, less aggressive chemo course.

"Psychologically, fasting was extremely helpful to me. The 'story' of my treatment seems fairly coherent when summarized, but when you are living through it, it feels like you are lurching from one course to another, with setbacks and unexpected additional treatments being thrown at you, as well as excruciating waits for results," A.P. said. "For me, fasting was something that allowed me to feel a bit more in control of my treatment."

When it came time for the stem cell transplant, she also fasted, and she finally finished her treatment in the summer of 2016 with 80 percent tumor reduction, demoting the cancer to stage III.

Stefano Quintarelli

Stefano is an entrepreneur and former professor of information systems, network services, and security.

"On a Friday in January 2018, I went to see my hematologist and he told me, 'It is leukemia, but don't worry, I will see you next week and will explain everything.' The expression *don't worry* associated with the word *leukemia* was really an oxymoron.

"A few months prior, during dinner, I heard that Valter was conducting promising animal studies on the effects of fasting and the fasting-mimicking diet on different types of leukemia. So I called him in Los Angeles. He told me that there was a trial that had recently started in a couple of Italian hospitals. I went to the National Cancer Institute in Milan, where I was enrolled in an experimental protocol that involved the use of a fasting-mimicking diet in patients with onco-hematological diseases.

"I now follow the Longevity Diet with a limited intake of carbohydrates. I continue to fast, always under medical supervision, but less frequently, depending on the progress of my hematological tests.

"The result is that more than six years after the diagnosis, my condition has remained stable, and I have not had to take *any* cancer drugs. Of course, there is no counterproof that the fasting-mimicking diet helped stabilize my disease. So my case, taken alone, cannot be considered statistically significant and exportable to other patients, nor is it possible to state with certainty how the evolution of my disease would have been if I had not cyclically carried out the fasting-mimicking diet.

"However, together with the data from preclinical studies, my case provides encouraging data that suggest further clinical studies are needed to evaluate the real clinical benefit provided by the fasting-mimicking diet in patients suffering from a disease like mine. In the meantime, the experimental path I have carried out has allowed me to avoid traditional immunosuppressive or myelosuppressive treatments, like chemotherapy, up to now. And that is very good for me."

BLOOD CANCER TREATMENT SUMMARY

- Follow standard cancer therapy (chemotherapy, etc.).
- Talk to your oncologist about combining standard therapy with the fasting-mimicking diet or, if standard therapy is not needed, about adopting a fasting-mimicking diet and possibly an extended seven-day version of the fasting-mimicking diet every two months.
- Between treatments, and for "watch and wait" patients in the absence of other treatments, follow the Longevity Diet (see chapter 3).
- Fast for thirteen to fourteen hours a day (for example, eating only between 8:00 a.m. and 6:00 p.m.) during the therapy, making sure to maintain normal muscle mass.
- Maintain a normal body weight.
- Be physically active and exercise, after consulting with your oncologist.
- Try to keep your phase angle (an indicator of muscular function) above 5 by doing strength training at least three or four times a week for thirty to forty minutes; you can follow the exercise video on the Create Cures website's section "Exercise and Longevity."

I DEDICATE THIS CHAPTER TO Woody Wright and to his courage in fighting a long battle with cancer, using everything his and my laboratories had learned about aging and cancer.

Patients who would like to learn more about the fasting/nutrition-based interventions described in this chapter should contact the Longevity and Healthspan Clinic of the Create Cures Foundation.

10

FASTING, NUTRITION, AND BRAIN CANCER

For their contributions and revisions to this chapter, I thank Thomas Chen, MD, surgical neuro-oncology director of the Brain and Spine Tumor Research Group and professor of neurological surgery, pathology, and orthopedic surgery at USC's Keck School of Medicine in Los Angeles; Fernando Safdie, MD, thoracic and foregut surgeon in the Division of Cardiothoracic Surgery at Mount Sinai Medical Center in Miami; Alessandro Laviano, MD, associate professor of medicine in the Department of Translational and Precision Medicine at Sapienza University of Rome; and Lizzia Raffaghello, PhD researcher in biology at the Giannina Gaslini Institute in Genoa.

BRAIN CANCER: WHAT IT IS AND HOW IT IS TREATED

Every year, about 30 people out of 100,000 are affected by brain cancer. Gliomas are the most frequent type, representing up to 78 percent of malignant brain tumors.[1]

Astrocytoma is the most common glioma. It originates from astrocytes, which are cells that form tissues that surround and protect nerve cells in the brain and spinal cord.

Ependymomas arise from ependymal cells, which form the inner lining of the ventricles of the brain.

Oligodendrogliomas arise from cells that wrap around nerve cells, forming an insulating sheath that facilitates nerve impulse conduction.

Glioblastoma multiforme (grade IV) represents the most aggressive malignant glioma.

Neuroblastoma is a cancer of the nervous system that mainly appears in newborns and children. It originates in neuroblasts, early or developing brain cells present in the sympathetic nervous system.

Diagnosing brain cancers requires a combination of medical evaluation, clinical symptoms, and diagnostic imaging, including contrast-enhanced computed tomography (CT) and magnetic resonance imaging (MRI). Biopsies allow the characterization and definitive diagnosis of brain masses. When possible, surgery is the treatment of choice, while preserving, as much as possible, neurological function. Additional and/or supplemental therapies include before-surgery (neoadjuvant) or after-surgery (adjuvant) chemoradiotherapy. Radiation after surgery is recommended for incomplete removals of tumors.

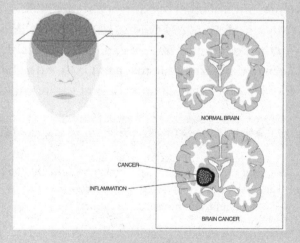

NORMAL BRAIN

CANCER

INFLAMMATION

BRAIN CANCER

10.1. *Tumors can start in early nerve cells (called neuroblasts) or other cells of the brain (glial cells). As a result, different types of tumors can form, and can be either benign or malignant.*

. . . .

IN 2012, WE PUBLISHED A study showing that neuroblastoma killed 100 percent of laboratory mice in sixty-five days, despite treatment with a potent, toxic chemotherapy agent. Yet mice treated with a combination of the same chemo agent and fasting demonstrated a 25 percent survival rate at one year, suggesting that they were likely free of cancer (in mice, these cancers are generally lethal within a few months). In a similar experiment (with a different type of neuroblastoma), mice treated with a combination of fasting and chemotherapy had an overall long-term survival rate of 42 percent, whereas the control group had 100 percent mortality by day 80 (figure 10.2).

The combination of chemotherapy and fasting has also shown promise with another type of cancer of the nervous system, glioblastoma. In this case, the cancer starts in the brain's glial cells, which provide support and protection to neurons. It was the cancer that claimed six-term U.S. senator and presidential candidate John McCain's life in 2018. By the time McCain was diagnosed with glioblastoma, we had been working with oncologists for ten years to test the combination of fasting and cancer therapies, but unfortunately, we did not have sufficient data to be able to recommend fasting-mimicking diets to McCain. Beau Biden, son of former president Joe Biden, also died of glioblastoma in 2015 after a five-year battle. These are famous examples of a problem touching millions of people. They reflect how the system is not optimal for patients with advanced-stage and aggressive disease, especially those who, like John McCain or Beau Biden, run out of viable options and could have been helped by our or other promising integrative interventions.

But we continue to do research in the hope of helping future cancer patients. In 2012, we published several papers showing that fasting cycles could make both chemotherapy and radiotherapy significantly more effective against this cancer in mice. One paper was from a study conducted by Dr. Fernando Safdie in my group,

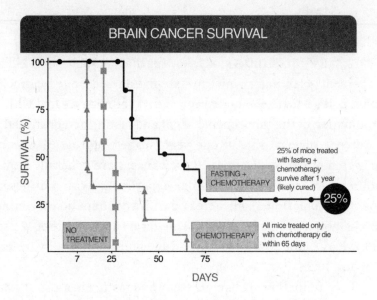

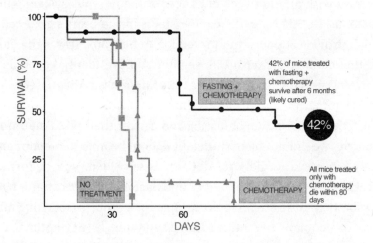

10.2. *Top graph: All mice with neuroblastoma treated with chemotherapy died within sixty-five days, while 25 percent of mice treated with chemotherapy and fasting were alive and likely free of cancer after one year. Bottom graph: All mice with neuroblastoma treated with chemotherapy died within eighty days, while 42 percent of mice treated with chemotherapy and fasting were alive and probably free of cancer after six months,. Modified from Changhan Lee et al., "Fasting Cycles Retard Growth of Tumors and Sensitize a Range of Cancer Cell Types to Chemotherapy,"* Science Translational Medicine *4, no. 124 (2012): 124ra27.*

. . . .

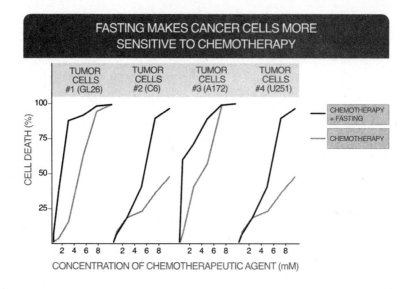

10.3. *When the concentration of chemotherapy drugs increases, so does the cell death of different types of glial cancer (i.e., cancer of the supporting cells in the central nervous system). The effect is stronger when chemotherapy is combined with fasting. Modified from Fernando Safdie et al., "Fasting Enhances the Response of Glioma to Chemo- and Radiotherapy,"* PLOS ONE *7, no. 9 (2012): e44603.*

who examined the benefits of fasting combined with the chemotherapy drug temozolomide (TMZ), and he found that, when combined with fasting, TMZ was significantly more effective in killing five different glioblastoma cancers taken from both humans and mice (figure 10.3). Notably, fasting conditions appeared to protect the normal cells while sensitizing the tumor cells to the drug.

A single cycle of fasting combined with chemotherapy was also very effective in delaying the growth of glioblastoma in mice, whereas chemotherapy alone had little effect on cancer growth. In fact, after one month, only 40 percent of mice treated with chemotherapy or fasting alone survived, versus 80 percent of those combining fasting and chemotherapy (figure 10.4).[2]

We observed similar effects when we combined fasting and radiotherapy in the treatment of glioblastoma. Fasting made radiotherapy more effective against cancer cells. After one month, 80

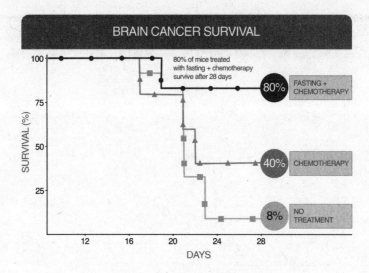

10.4. *Fasting made chemotherapy more effective against cancer cells, and after one month, 80 percent of mice were still alive, versus 40 percent of those that received chemotherapy alone. Modified from Fernando Safdie et al., "Fasting Enhances the Response of Glioma to Chemo- and Radiotherapy," PLOS ONE 7, no. 9 (2012): e44603.*

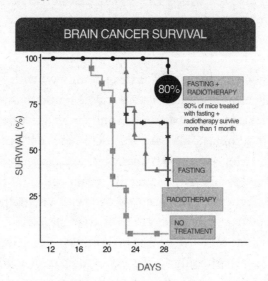

10.5. *Fasting made radiotherapy more effective against cancer cells. After one month, 80 percent of mice receiving both fasting and radiotherapy were alive, versus less than 40 percent survival for those receiving only radiotherapy or fasting. Modified from Fernando Safdie et al., "Fasting Enhances the Response of Glioma to Chemo- and Radiotherapy," PLOS ONE 7, no. 9 (2012): e44603.*

percent of mice receiving both fasting and radiotherapy were alive, versus fewer than 40 percent of those receiving radiotherapy or fasting alone (figure 10.5).

FASTING AND BRAIN CANCERS: KETOGENIC DIETS

The Warburg effect, explained in chapter 7, describes the changes in cancer cells leading to increased uptake and use of sugar by cancer cells. For this reason, I review recent studies testing ketogenic diets that are low in carbohydrates and their effectiveness against brain cancers in humans, since very few studies have yet looked at the role of fasting-mimicking diets on glioblastoma progression in humans.

As discussed earlier, ketogenic diets (1) are very high in fat and low in carbohydrates (usually with a 4:1 or higher ratio of fats to carbs), (2) can have either low-protein or high-protein content, and (3) provide a normal number of calories, but (4) are designed to be consumed every day for weeks to months or longer during cancer treatment. The fasting-mimicking diet has some similarities to the ketogenic diet in its high fat and relatively low carb content, but fasting-mimicking diets are also low in calories, very low in protein, and plant-based. Unlike ketogenic diets, fasting-mimicking diets are usually consumed for only four or five days a month (figure 10.6).

Since the ketogenic diet provides a normal level of calories, including calories from fat and proteins, it can either combat or favor cancer growth, depending on the cancer type. However, because glioblastomas are so aggressive, several animal studies indicate that a ketogenic diet can slow down the growth of this cancer. Further testing of the efficacy of the combination of ketogenic and fasting-mimicking diets with standard therapies is needed to understand the optimal use of nutritechnology against these cancers.

CHARACTERISTICS	KETOGENIC DIET	FASTING-MIMICKING DIET
Calorie intake	Normal	Low
Carbohydrate (% of calories)	Low	Low-medium
Fat intake (% of calories)	High	High
Protein intake	Ranging from moderate to high	Very low
Duration	Weeks to months	4–5 days every 3–8 weeks
Composition	Both animal- and plant-based	Plant-based

10.6. *A comparison between main features of the ketogenic diet and the fasting-mimicking diet.*

FASTING, THE KETOGENIC DIET, AND CLINICAL TRIALS

There have been a few clinical trials that studied the effects of the ketogenic diet with or without fasting on glioblastoma patients. In a 2020 study, a group of German clinicians tested the effect of a combination of a ketogenic diet plus water-only fasting. Glioblastoma patients received either (1) radiation and a healthy diet or (2) radiation plus a single cycle of six days of a ketogenic diet combined with three days of water-only fasting. The single nine-day dietary change did not make a significant difference in the glioblastoma's progression. After six months, 20 percent of the patients on a fasting/ketogenic diet combined with radiation had not progressed, versus 16 percent of those who received radiation only.[3]

This is not surprising, since only one cycle of the fasting and ketogenic diets was administered, and no effective drugs were used. A new trial is needed to test monthly cycles of the combination of fasting-mimicking diet with or without ketogenic diet plus standard treatments including radiation and chemotherapy. Because this cancer is very aggressive, the treatment must be more aggressive. Only multiple cycles of the fasting-mimicking diet (and potentially the ketogenic diet) together with standard drugs or new drugs that synergize with the fasting and radiation have a chance of making a difference in patients' survival.

This study provided very important information on the effect of blood glucose levels on the survival of patients with glioblastoma. In those patients who completed the fasting-and-ketogenic-diet cycle and reached blood glucose levels below 83.5 mg/dl, cancer clearly grew more slowly, and the patients survived longer, with 20 percent living for nearly three years, whereas none of those who had blood glucose levels above 83.5 mg/dl survived for more than thirteen months. Because we already know that fasting-mimicking-diet cycles lower glucose levels, these results underscore the need for monthly fasting-mimicking-diet cycles alternating with a low-protein, vegan ketogenic diet and the Longevity Diet, plus standard therapy—radiation and chemotherapy, or new cancer drugs such as immunotherapy—to fight brain cancer. Again, this is still an experimental and complex protocol, which was carried out by the Create Cures Foundation clinic on several brain cancer patients in coordination with their oncologists. Several have had excellent results thus far, but large clinical trials must be conducted. If a patient were to do this, it should be under the supervision of a multipronged team including an oncologist, a molecular biologist, and a nutritionist who has experience in ketogenic diets and fasting-mimicking diets.

In 2011, a case report describing the use of fasting along with a ketogenic diet in brain cancer treatment was published. It discussed the case of a sixty-five-year-old woman with multicentric glioblastoma multiforme (GBM), a highly malignant cancer belonging to the astrocytoma class. In the beginning, she was treated with the standard therapy, a three-day water-only therapeutic fast and a fourteen-day restricted ketogenic diet with a 4:1 ratio of fat to carbohydrate and protein that delivered about six hundred calories per day, supplemented with vitamins and minerals, for two cycles. However, due to hyperuricemia (an accumulation of the waste product uric acid in the blood, which can cause kidney stones), the second cycle of a calorie-restricted diet was nonketogenic.[4] The patient responded well to dietary therapy, and after two months of treatment, her cancer was no longer visible by imaging techniques such as PET or MRI. Ten weeks after discontinuing the dietary therapy, however, her cancer returned.

In 2018, a case report of a thirty-eight-year-old man with glioblastoma multiforme (GBM) was published in *Frontiers in Nutrition*. The patient had been treated with a modified standard of care (surgery, radiotherapy, and chemotherapy) together with a ketogenic diet and fasting. The patient fasted for seventy-two hours prior to surgical removal of the tumor. After fasting, he followed a calorie-restricted (900 calories per day) ketogenic / high-protein fasting-mimicking diet for twenty-one days, supplemented with vitamins and minerals. At day 22, the calories of this ketogenic diet were increased to 1,500 per day, and the patient also received hyperbaric oxygen therapy (breathing pure oxygen in a pressurized environment) and other targeted metabolic therapies. Clinical analysis revealed a therapeutic benefit of presurgical metabolic therapy (thanks to the ketogenic / fasting-mimicking diet), and the patient remained in excellent health with continued evidence of significant tumor regression for at least two years.[5]

ONE SMALL 2014 CLINICAL TRIAL in twenty adult patients with recurrent glioblastoma multiforme showed that the ketogenic diet is feasible, even if it was low in compliance and poorly tolerated, so the results were not statistically significant. Moreover, the ketogenic diet is not recommended as a unique therapy (used without standard of care therapy) and should be evaluated by the oncologist.[6]

Other results were published in 2015 by a research group from Michigan State University. It included case reports of two glioma patients who went on an energy-restricted ketogenic diet as their only form of therapy, and, unfortunately, the cancer progressed. In contrast, these researchers also reported findings on thirty patients from other case reports and clinical trials who were treated with an assortment of ketogenic diet protocols in combination with standard therapies (of the thirty patients, only one was treated with the ketogenic diet as the only therapy). They showed prolonged remission, i.e., no signs of cancer, for periods ranging from four months to more than five years, with no major side effects.[7]

In 2017, a randomized pilot study was published on the impact on twelve patients' health and quality of life of a ketogenic diet as an additional therapy, given after their primary treatment for glioblastoma.[8] The results showed that recruitment and retention were low, as only four of twelve patients completed the three-month diet. There were no results in cancer progression, since this study was focused on whether patients could complete the diet.[9]

Because of the keto diet's rigid food recommendations, compliance has been proving a major issue. Researchers in the Netherlands published a 2019 analysis regarding eleven glioblastoma multiforme patients who followed a liquid ketogenic diet for six weeks, starting two weeks before the first cycle of chemotherapy or radiation. After six weeks, the diet was modified to include solid foods and additional calories from coconut oil–derived medium-chain triglycerides. This ketogenic diet was followed for a total period of fourteen weeks. Of the eleven patients, nine reached ketosis and six completed the study, with no severe adverse effects. It emerged that the ketogenic diet was feasible for patients, but a supportive partner and intensive counseling is essential for compliance.[10]

In order to aid in this challenge, researchers from Bethesda, Maryland, developed a novel 4:1 ketogenic-diet approach (four parts fats and one part proteins and carbohydrates). This pilot study evaluated feasibility, safety, tolerability, and efficacy for glioblastoma multiforme for six months. Of eight patients, five completed the six months, while three subjects stopped because of either glioblastoma multiforme progression or diet restrictiveness. Unfortunately, because of the small sample size of the study, it is not possible to reach definitive conclusions, even if the diet appeared to be well tolerated.[11]

As reported, most of these studies provide data only on feasibility and short-term safety, since most of the trials are nonrandomized (there is no comparison between two different groups), are short term, and involve advanced-stage cancer patients. It is clear that randomized clinical studies are necessary to further evaluate the potential therapeutic role, effectiveness, safety, and feasibility of ketogenic diets targeting brain cancer.

PATIENTS' STORIES AND EXPERIENCES

Sebastien

In 2019, Sebastien was forty-eight and worked as a research scientist for a multinational corporation. One day, biking home from work, he took a wrong turn and felt disoriented; it surprised him, as he had taken the same route every day for more than fifteen years. A couple of weeks later, he bumped into tables and chairs in a restaurant, and the next day he woke up with a severe headache.

Soon after, Sebastien visited his doctor, and after some tests, he was diagnosed with stage IV brain cancer. Five days later he had surgery, and most of the visible cancer was removed. Six weeks later, he started radiation treatments and chemotherapy, but the glioblastoma did not respond well to treatment. He remembers, "As I felt my world collapsing, my resolve to fight this with everything I had increased."

Sebastien bought books on cancer, nutrition, and meditation and searched scientific papers for everything on glioblastoma. One friend forwarded him a podcast with one of my interviews explaining the fasting-mimicking diet and how it was a hopeful tool in fighting cancer. Encouraged, Sebastien found the study that showed the fasting-mimicking diet, in tandem with standard chemo treatment (temozolomide, or TMZ), had positive results for glioblastoma in rodents.

After he read this article, he decided to fast during the five days of chemotherapy every month. "My first few months of chemotherapy, without the fasting-mimicking diet, were tolerable, but by the fourth or the fifth day I became very tired. Undergoing chemotherapy while fasting changed my perspective. I was not just reducing the side effects of the standard treatment but taking charge. I am not going to say that I enjoyed the five days of fasting / fasting-mimicking diet, but I could function normally and was not bedridden," Sebastien says.

An MRI shortly after starting his first fasting-mimicking diet showed a 50 percent reduction in the size of the abnormal brain tissue, and his MRI was clear by the end of the six months of TMZ treatment, the last two concurrent with the fasting-mimicking diet.

Fifteen months post operation, he was back to work at 80 percent. He continues the fasting-mimicking diet, once every two months, hoping that it will help prevent the cancer from returning.

Marianna Incorvaia

"My mother, who was seventy in September of 2020, seemed exhausted and weak after a family vacation. In October, she started to have speech difficulties and was forgetting names of objects and people. When it got worse, I talked to our family doctor, who ordered her an MRI. It showed that she had a glioblastoma.

"Neurosurgeons at the University Hospital in Bern told us that surgery was not possible. Instead, they had her start a six-week radiotherapy cycle combined with chemotherapy treatment with a daily intake of the drug Temodal. Radiotherapy had devastating effects on her. She struggled to control her emotions and behaved irrationally at times. During the second half of this cycle, she suffered from severe fatigue and hunger, but she was also on a high dosage of cortisone, which made it impossible to follow any major dietary change.

"The six-week cycle was followed by a four-week break, which my mom largely spent sleeping up to twenty hours a day. She no longer existed. She no longer had irrational moments, but she barely communicated and was apathetic.

"After this four-week break, she started with a five-day chemotherapy cycle with a higher Temodal dosage. During which, she also followed a five-day fasting-mimicking diet. We had already read a lot about Professor Valter Longo's research, and we had also fasted before then. And although we were optimistic, we did not expect such a surprising outcome.

"This cycle of chemotherapy combined with the fasting-mimicking diet had enormous effects. At the end of these five days, we had our mom back. She was present, awake, and communicating with us. She seemed to understand what was happening to her and she was able to express her emotions again. Fatigue decreased considerably. After another cycle of chemo and fast-mimicking diet, she continued to feel better and more energetic. After the third cycle of chemo and the third cycle of a fasting-mimicking diet, Mom's recovery was notable, especially physically. Because of the cortisone she had to take, Mom had developed a form of diabetes, but during the cycles of the fasting-mimicking diet she did not need any insulin.

"I believe that my mom was able to recover due to the combination of these various treatments. Without the fasting-mimicking diet, I believe the situation today would be much worse."

Kevin

In January 2018, Kevin, an American living in China, was diagnosed with an inoperable oligodendroglioma mixed with astrocytoma. Searching for additional cures or therapies other than the standard radiation/chemotherapy cocktail, he came across our research, and he adopted the fasting regime (with some difficulty fasting for more than two days in the beginning) and practiced intermittent fasting (IF) in between longer-term fasts.

The most important result has been a 50 percent reduction of his cancer and complete disappearance of the metastasis. Moreover, his new dietary habits completely changed his overall health, once he also adopted an everyday nutrition regime similar to the Longevity Diet.

"To say that Professor Longo's research has saved my life is an understatement," he says. "He has given me my health back, but also the opportunity to enjoy a longer and happier life with my three children and to impact their lives for the better, too. For that, I am eternally grateful."

BRAIN CANCER TREATMENT SUMMARY

- Follow standard cancer therapy (chemotherapy, radiation, etc.).
- Talk to your oncologist about combining standard therapy with a fasting-mimicking diet.
- Talk to your oncologist and a nutritionist in order to combine the fasting-mimicking diet with a plant-and-fish-based ketogenic diet low in protein; make sure it does not negatively affect body weight.
- Between treatments, follow the Longevity Diet (see chapter 3).
- Fast for fourteen hours a day (for example, eating only between 8:00 a.m. and 6:00 p.m.).
- Maintain a normal body weight.
- Be physically active and exercise, after consulting your oncologist.
- Try to keep your phase angle (an indicator of muscular function) above 5 by doing strength training at least three or four times a week for thirty to forty minutes; you can

follow the exercise video on the Create Cures website's section "Exercise and Longevity."

Patients who would like to learn more about the fasting/nutrition-based interventions described in this chapter should contact the Longevity and Healthspan Clinic of the Create Cures Foundation.

11

FASTING, NUTRITION, AND SKIN CANCER

For their contributions and revisions to this chapter, I thank Christian Posch, MD, PhD, head of the Department of Dermatology at Vienna Healthcare Group, Austria; and Alessandro Laviano, MD, associate professor of medicine in the Department of Translational and Precision Medicine at Sapienza University of Rome.

SKIN CANCER: WHAT IT IS AND HOW TO TREAT IT

Melanoma is a type of skin cancer. According to the World Cancer Research Fund and the American Institute for Cancer Research, it is the seventeenth-most-common cancer, with nearly 325,000 cases in 2020 worldwide.[1] The risk of melanoma typically increases as we age, but people in every age group can develop it. Melanoma predominantly affects fair-skinned people: the lifetime risk of developing melanoma is estimated to be one in fifty for Caucasians. There are two different types of skin tumors:

1. **Epithelioma** originates from lining cells called keratinocytes.

2. **Melanoma** originates from melanocytes, responsible for the production of melanin, the pigment for skin and hair color present at the junction of superficial and deep layers of the skin.

The most frequent site of onset is the trunk (back, chest, head, and neck) in men and limbs (especially legs) in women, while it can also originate from melanocytes in the eyes, although this is rare.

In recent decades, the incidence of cutaneous melanoma in the Caucasian population has grown by 3 to 5 percent every year.

Early-stage tumors can effectively be treated surgically, with a cure rate of more than 98 percent in stage IA disease, but if the cancer has a thickness of more than one millimeter, it will require an examination of the sentinel lymph node (the lymph node nearest the skin area where a melanoma has been diagnosed). Local radiotherapy is also used to reduce the risk of recurrence. For advanced, systemic disease, immunotherapy and kinase-targeted therapies have almost completely replaced chemotherapy, as they have proven to be more effective.[2]

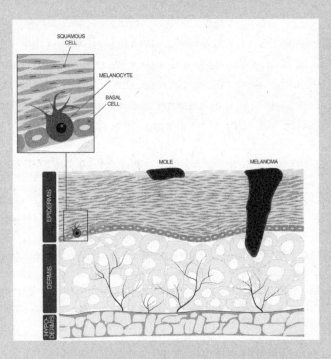

11.1. *Cutaneous melanoma is a cancer that results from the transformation of melanocytes, a type of skin cell. The main sign of skin melanoma is a change in the appearance of a mole or if a new mole with special features appears. The vast majority of moles are benign, but melanomas often have asymmetrical shapes, poorly defined borders, and different colors. They can also change in size—most become larger than a quarter of an inch (about six millimeters)—and shape.*

· · · · · · ·

AROUND 2018, I PARTICIPATED IN a meeting with some of the leading cancer researchers and clinicians. One of the oncologists, who played a central role in the demonstration of the efficacy of immunotherapy against melanoma, told the story of how the first key trial on immunotherapy and melanoma almost ended up being viewed as a failure, since it did not show significant effects on the entire population tested, although it worked well on a portion of that population. A few years later, based in large part on the clinical success of immunotherapy against melanoma, the 2018 Nobel Prize in Physiology or Medicine was awarded to the scientists who had first described immunotherapy drugs that can make the immune system more aggressive against melanoma cancer cells (figure 11.2)

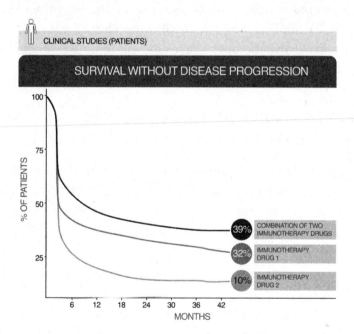

11.2. *The combination of medicines used for immunotherapy makes the immune system much more aggressive against melanoma cells and has an extraordinary effect on patient survival forty-two months after the beginning of the treatment. Modified from Jedd D. Wolchok et al., "Overall Survival with Combined Nivolumab and Ipilimumab in Advanced Melanoma,"* New England Journal of Medicine *377, no. 14 (2017): 1345–56.*

The original trial on melanoma immunotherapy worked well on only a relatively small portion of patients. In addition to this limitation, the cost of immunotherapy is extremely high—it can be more than $100,000 per year for a single patient. Two years earlier we had published on how the much less expensive fasting-mimicking diet, in combination with chemotherapy, could work like immunotherapy in mice and make the immune cells much more aggressive against melanoma as well as against breast cancer cells. Naturally, large clinical trials demonstrating the immune effects of the fasting-mimicking diet remain to be performed, and at the time of publication of this book we are continuing to investigate two questions: (1) Can the fasting-mimicking diet make immunotherapy more effective and increase the type and portion of responding patients? (2) Is it possible to use the fasting-mimicking diet in combination with other inexpensive drugs to mimic the effects of immunotherapy for people who cannot afford this extremely expensive therapy? I am cautiously optimistic about both.

FASTING, FASTING-MIMICKING DIET, AND SKIN CANCERS: LABORATORY STUDIES

Our first study to treat melanoma did not use fasting specifically but included mice that had a major reduction of IGF-1, an effect that is also key for the efficacy of fasting against many cancers. One group had normal levels of IGF-1 and another had very low levels of IGF-1. We treated mice with cycles of chemotherapy (doxorubicin), and after sixty days, 100 percent of the normal mice had died from either the cancer or the side effects of the chemotherapy, whereas 60 percent of the mice with low IGF-1 were alive, even after ninety days (figure 11.3). Cancer therapy alone can delay cancer growth, but when combined with very low IGF-1 levels (which are reduced by the fasting), it can become much more effective and can even cure a portion of mice of melanoma.

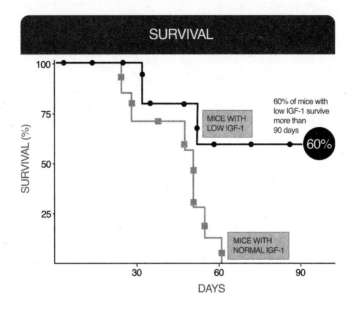

11.3. *After sixty days of chemotherapy, all mice with normal levels of IGF-1 (growth factor) had died. In contrast, 60 percent of the mice with low IGF-1 were alive even after ninety days, suggesting that they were cancer free. Modified from Changhan Lee et al., "Reduced Levels of IGF-I Mediate Differential Protection of Normal and Cancer Cells in Response to Fasting and Improve Chemotherapeutic Index,"* Cancer Research *70, no. 4 (2010): 1564–72.*

We saw similar results when we injected melanoma cancer cells into mice that had very low IGF-1 because of the genetic mutation GHRD (a mutation similar to those in Ecuadorians with Laron syndrome, who are rarely affected by tumors) (figure 11.4, bottom graph) and into mice whose IGF-1 was lowered by feeding them a very low-protein diet (figure 11.4, top graph).[3]

A few years later we combined fasting with chemotherapy (doxorubicin or cyclophosphamide) for the treatment of melanoma, and we observed a major delay in cancer growth but did not see any mice being cured (figure 11.5). One possible explanation for this is that these drugs are not commonly used to treat melanoma. Therefore, as mentioned in previous chapters, matching the most

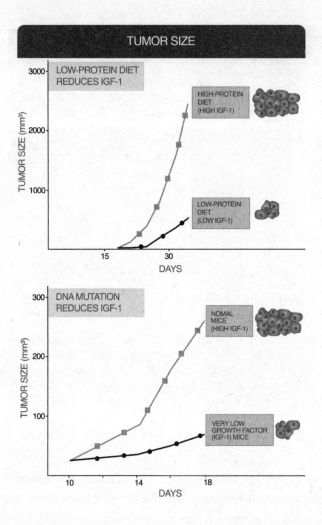

11.4. *Top graph: Melanoma tumors grow to a larger size in mice fed with a high-protein diet. Bottom graph: Melanoma tumors remain smaller in mice that have very low levels of IGF-1 because of a genetic mutation (GHRD) than in normal mice. Modified from Morgan E. Levine et al., "Low Protein Intake Is Associated with a Major Reduction in IGF-1, Cancer, and Overall Mortality in the 65 and Younger but Not Older Population,"* Cell Metabolism *19, no. 3 (March 4, 2014): 407–17.*

effective drug against a particular cancer with fasting-mimicking diet cycles seems to cause a stronger effect and potentially cancer-free survival.[4]

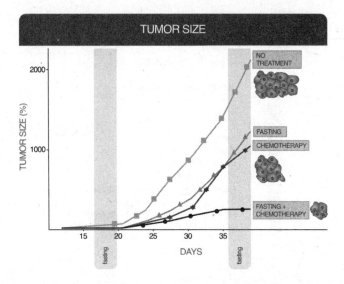

11.5. *Melanoma growth in mice is delayed, thanks to fasting and chemotherapy. However, mice do not become cancer free. Modified from Hong Seok Shim et al., "Starvation Promotes REV1 SUMOylation and p53-Dependent Sensitization of Melanoma and Breast Cancer Cells,"* Cancer Research 75, no. 6 (2015): 1056–67.

Although the combination of chemotherapy and fasting did not result in cured mice, it delayed cancer growth and reduced metastasis of melanoma cells in the kidneys, lymph nodes, ovaries, spleen, and liver (figure 11.6).[5]

To better understand how fasting makes chemotherapy more effective against melanoma, we conducted an experiment examining DNA damage in melanoma cancer cells treated with chemotherapy alone or with chemotherapy plus fasting. The level of DNA damage in the melanoma cells was around 2 (in a range from 0 to 60) without treatment; it remained 2 after chemotherapy. It reached 6 with fasting alone but increased to 40 when chemotherapy was combined with fasting (figure 11.7).[6]

At the time of the publication of this book, we are combining fasting-mimicking diets in animal and clinical trials with drugs other than chemotherapy, including drugs that lower the levels of

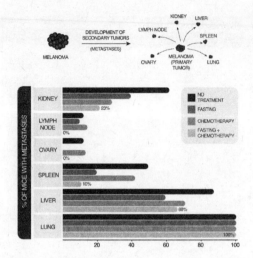

11.6. *A forty-eight-hour fast combined with chemotherapy reduced the metastasis of melanoma cells in kidneys, lymph nodes, ovaries, spleen, and liver, although it did not lead to mice's cancer-free survival. Modified from Changhan Lee et al., "Fasting Cycles Retard Growth of Tumors and Sensitize a Range of Cancer Cell Types to Chemotherapy,"* Science Translational Medicine *4, no. 124 (2012): 124ra27.*

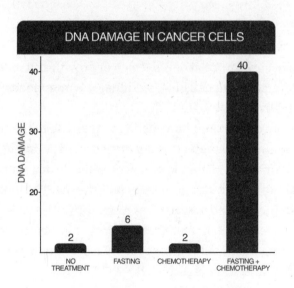

11.7. *Levels of DNA damage in melanoma cancer cells treated with chemotherapy alone or combined with fasting. Modified from Changhan Lee et al., "Fasting Cycles Retard Growth of Tumors and Sensitize a Range of Cancer Cell Types to Chemotherapy,"* Science Translational Medicine *4, no. 124 (2012): 124ra27.*

IGF-1. The purpose is to force cancer cells into the most hostile conditions possible without negatively affecting normal cells. Since we know that people on the fasting-mimicking diet show a reduction in IGF-1, we can surmise that the combination of drugs lowering IGF-1, fasting-mimicking diets, plus standard-of-care cancer drugs have the potential to be effective in the treatment of multiple cancers, by being lethal to cancer cells and beneficial to normal cells and organs.

It will be important to test the combination of fasting / fasting-mimicking diet, IGF-1–lowering drugs, and drugs targeting the cancer specifically, such as immunotherapy, kinase inhibitors, and other cutting-edge treatments as they are developed.

CAN FASTING REPLACE IMMUNOTHERAPY OR MAKE IT WORK BETTER?

Fasting-mimicking-diet cycles rejuvenate the immune system and reduce tumor size in mice, which could indicate that more functional and more aggressive immune cells contribute to the effects of fasting against cancer cells.[7] Motivated by this, we looked at whether the fasting-mimicking diet could stimulate the immune system to attack melanoma cells. As observed with breast cancer, when we treated mice with melanoma with either the fasting-mimicking diet or chemotherapy (doxorubicin) alone, we saw a small increase in the number of immune cells attacking the cancer, but when we combined chemotherapy and fasting-mimicking diet cycles, the attack on the cancer by the immune cells increased threefold (figure 11.8), resulting in tumors that were three times smaller than those in the untreated mice (figure 11.9).

Another laboratory study treated human melanoma cells in the lab with either fasting alone, a kinase inhibitor cancer drug (Sorafenib), or both. In the first two groups, they saw either little or no effect on melanoma cells, but the combination of fasting and the kinase inhibitor killed nearly all of two different types of

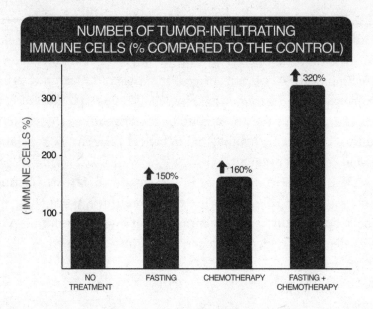

11.8. *Mice with melanoma treated with either a fasting-mimicking diet or chemotherapy alone showed a small increase in the number of immune cells attacking the cancer mass. However, when chemotherapy and fasting-mimicking-diet cycles were combined, the attack against cancer masses by the immune cells increased threefold. Modified from Stefano Di Biase et al., "Fasting-Mimicking Diet Reduces HO-1 to Promote T Cell–Mediated Tumor Cytotoxicity," Cancer Cell 30, no. 1 (July 11, 2016): 136–46.*

melanoma cells. Once again, the drug or fasting alone did little to kill cancer cells, but in combination they were highly effective.[8]

FASTING, FASTING-MIMICKING DIET, AND CANCER TREATMENT: CLINICAL STUDIES

Although we have not yet carried out a clinical trial on melanoma and fasting-mimicking diets, a number of patients have combined the fasting / fasting-mimicking diet with other therapies as part of several ongoing clinical trials. In one published study, the authors looked at the patients' levels of leptin, which regulates glucose levels, and the role of diabetes in patients with melanoma to see how they were affected. Patients with high levels of leptin had a higher

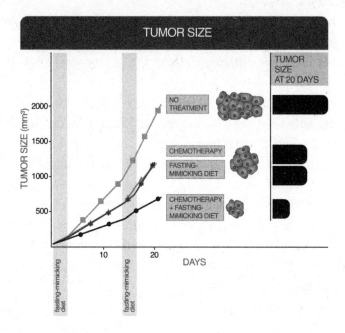

11.9. *The melanoma mass of mice treated with combined chemotherapy fasting-mimicking-diet cycles are three times smaller than those in the untreated mice. Modified from Stefano Di Biase et al., "Fasting-Mimicking Diet Reduces HO-1 to Promote T Cell–Mediated Tumor Cytotoxicity," Cancer Cell 30, no. 1 (July 11, 2016): 136–46.*

chance of melanoma metastases than those with lower leptin levels. In addition, melanoma patients with diabetes had reduced life expectancy.[9]

MELANOMA TREATMENT SUMMARY

- Follow standard cancer therapy (immunotherapy, kinase inhibitors, etc).
- Talk to your oncologist about combining standard therapy with a fasting-mimicking diet, especially in advanced-stage cancers with poor prognosis.
- If this is not sufficient, talk to an oncologist and a nutritionist in order to combine a fasting-mimicking diet

with a ketogenic diet (low in protein and plant-and-fish-based).

- Between treatments, follow the Longevity Diet (see chapter 3).
- Fast for thirteen to fourteen hours a day (for example, eating only between 8:00 a.m. and 6:00 p.m.) during therapy.
- Maintain a normal body weight.
- Be physically active and exercise, after consulting an oncologist.
- Try to keep your phase angle (an indicator of muscular function) above 5 by doing strength training at least three or four times a week for thirty to forty minutes; you can follow the exercise video on the Create Cures website's section "Exercise and Longevity."

Patients who would like to learn more about the fasting/nutrition-based interventions described in this chapter should contact the Longevity and Healthspan Clinic of the Create Cures Foundation.

12

FASTING, NUTRITION, AND KIDNEY CANCER

For their review of this chapter, I thank Bernard Escudier, MD, former chair of the Renal Cancer Unit at the Gustave Roussy Institute in Villejuif, France, and former coordinator of the ESMO Kidney Cancer Advisory Group; and Alessandro Laviano, MD, associate professor of medicine in the Department of Translational and Precision Medicine at Sapienza University of Rome.

KIDNEY CANCER: WHAT IT IS AND HOW IT IS TREATED

Kidney cancer, also known as renal cancer, includes several types of cancer. Particularly in adults, it can consist of renal-cell carcinoma (RCC), the most common form, which appears in the largest part of the kidney (cortex and medulla), and renal transitional-cell carcinoma (RTCC), which originates in the renal pelvis (figure 12.1).

Kidney cancer is very common, with more than 430,000 new cases in the world in 2020, and is the ninth-most-common tumor in men and the fourteenth-most-common in women.[1]

Because the organ filters blood, the kidney is often exposed to toxins present in food, beverages, the environment, etc., all of which can contribute to the development of cancer.

Another risk factor is cigarette smoking, with the level of risk depending on the number of cigarettes smoked per day and the number of years spent smoking. Other risk factors include obesity, hypertension, reduced physical activity, high alcohol consumption, occupational exposure to chemical substances like trichloroethylene (used as a solvent in industrial work), and genetics. For women, having five or more pregnancies is also a risk factor.[2]

Renal tumors do not have clear clinical manifestations but can cause symptoms such as weakness, rapid and unjustified weight loss, and low-grade fever. As the disease progresses, more specific symptoms can include blood in the urine (hematuria), pain, and a renal mass that a doctor can feel during a medical examination.[3]

When a doctor suspects kidney cancer, the patient should have an ultrasound and a computed tomography (CT) scan, an MRI, and/or a urograph, a specific test to evaluate the urinary tract.

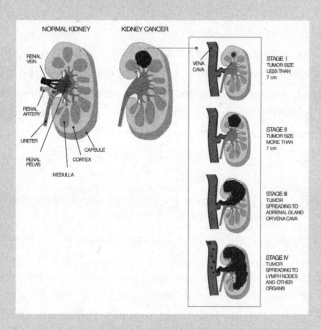

12.1. Renal-cell carcinoma (RCC), the most common form of kidney cancer, originates in the largest part of the kidney (cortex and medulla), while renal transitional-cell carcinoma (RTCC) develops in the renal pelvis. In stages I and II, the cancer is limited to the kidney, though in stage II it is larger. Stage III indicates it has extended to the lymph nodes nearby. In stage IV, the cancer extends outside of the kidneys, into lymph nodes or other sites including the bones, spleen, and/or lungs.

> If the cancer is localized and detected early, it can be surgi-
> cally removed. In many cases, surgery removes only the cancer,
> preserving the rest of the organ.
>
> Unfortunately, early diagnosis is difficult, and 25 to 30 percent
> of cases are at an advanced stage by the time they are detected,
> typically with distant metastases, especially in the lymph nodes,
> lungs, skeleton, liver, and other kidney. Moreover, cancer recur-
> rence can occur after surgery.
>
> Some kidney cancers are treated with nonchemotherapeutic
> drugs to inhibit angiogenesis, the process by which blood vessels
> are formed. Immunotherapy is also used. These therapies can also
> be combined to improve the patient's response.[4]

IN THE SPRING OF 2014, airline pilot Jean-Jacques Trochon was
told by his oncologist (Dr. Bernard Escudier of the Gustave Roussy
Institute) that he had a stage IV kidney cancer and needed to undergo urgent treatment for metastatic kidney tumors, which were
growing rapidly in his lungs. Dr. Escudier also told him about a
new (at the time) antiangiogenic therapy, focused on blocking the
supply of blood to the cancer, for which there was no evidence of
long-term patient survival. Jean-Jacques knew that if he accepted,
in addition to the uncertainty about whether it would work, this
treatment would mean the end of his flying career, based on airline rules. Instead, he convinced the hospital to perform a double
thoracotomy—a brutal surgical procedure whereby the chest cavity is opened through the rib cage and the metastases are removed
from the lungs. His oncologist believed that the patient was merely
putting off the inevitable and that the cancer would unavoidably
come back.

Jean-Jacques had also heard about fasting and cancer treatment from a 2012 French documentary entitled *Le jeûne: Une nou-
velle thérapie?* (Fasting: A new therapy?), which included my
interview. Excited by what he saw, he decided that fasting could be
the "missing link" he needed to fight the cancer ahead of surgery.
He contacted me and told me about his impending thoracotomies,
and while I recommended that he talk to his oncologist about

trying multiple shorter fasting-mimicking diet periods, he decided to undergo a twelve-day water fast. During the fast, Jean-Jacques was in regular contact with me as well as under the supervision of his doctor. After the anticipated difficulty of the initial few days, by day five he told me he was experiencing a sense of alertness and a surge in energy. By day nine, he was able to run several laps around the lake near his house. After the fast, the results were better than Jean-Jacques had hoped for: a preoperation scan showed that not only was there no further cancer growth, but also five of the ten cancers in his right lung had undergone necrosis (cell death), meaning many cancer masses were no longer visible or were not growing. Jean-Jacques told me that his surgeon had never seen anything like it before. Still, his surgeon worried about the twelve-day water fast, since it could put him in danger during the surgery by weakening his immune system. His oncologist felt the chance of remission was extremely low, even after the successful surgery, considering what the publications on this tumor reported.

Convinced of the benefits of fasting, Jean-Jacques decided to make it part of his personal protocol. In addition to many long fasting periods, he began intermittent fasting on a daily basis, eating his last meal no later than 8:00 p.m., skipping breakfast, and eating lunch around twelve o'clock the following day (sixteen hours daily fasting).

Soon Jean-Jacques felt better, and he returned to his airline career. He adopted the fasting-mimicking diet when flying, since it made him feel more alert. The news of Jean-Jacques's remarkable recovery spread among his airline colleagues. Impressed by his energy levels, many followed his example and adopted the fasting-mimicking-diet approach.

After retiring from Air France in 2020, Jean-Jacques continues to fight cancer, but ten years after the stage IV cancer diagnosis the masses remaining are either stable or calcified. Fasting approximately five days every month remains part of Jean-Jacques's central approach to a healthy life. Together with his wife, Heather Whitehall-Trochon, he wrote *Flying Against the Odds*, a memoir detailing his personal cancer journey.

LABORATORY RESEARCH

When you read about Jean-Jacques's initial success with a twelve-day water fast, it is easy to think that fasting can cure kidney cancer. Unfortunately, this is not the case. A laboratory at the University of Texas showed that long-term and severe calorie restriction had only a minor effect on kidney cancer growth in mice, unless it was combined with the blocking of autophagy, a type of cell self-cannibalism that occurs in response to starvation (figure 12.2).[5] More research is needed to understand how fasting-mimicking diets can be combined with standard or novel therapies to fight kidney cancer. Clearly, for someone like Jean-Jacques, with a very poor prognosis, fasting-mimicking-diet cycles in combination with standard therapy should be considered in consultation with an oncologist.

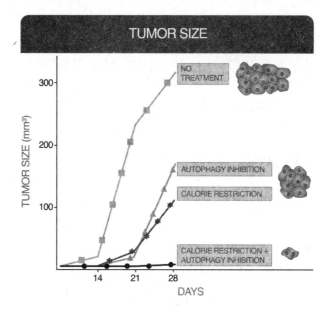

12.2. *Inhibition of autophagy (cells' ability to obtain energy by feeding off their own components, in a process similar to self-cannibalism), combined with calorie restriction, reduces kidney cancer growth in mice. Modified from Laura M. Lashinger et al., "Starving Cancer from the Outside and Inside: Separate and Combined Effects of Calorie Restriction and Autophagy Inhibition on Ras-Driven Tumors,"* Cancer Metabolism, *4, no. 18 (September 2016).*

· · · · · · ·

I HAVE SHOWN THROUGHOUT THE book that fasting and the fasting-mimicking diet act as an anticancer wild card; by pushing the tumor into a corner, it forces the cancer to try to find "escape routes." In the study above, that escape route was the ability of the cancer cells to get energy through autophagy. Fasting and drugs that inhibit autophagy work very well together to block all escape routes. Blocking autophagy with a drug may work for one type but not another type of kidney cancer, which may instead be more affected by lowering another starvation escape pathway, etc. In most situations, the fasting-mimicking diet can serve as an effective wild card, working best if combined with drugs that target the cellular pathways that allow cancer cells to escape and survive. In many cases, this can potentially be achieved by combining the standard of care (chemotherapy, hormone therapy, immunotherapy, etc.) with the fasting-mimicking diet. In other cases, it will be necessary to first apply the fasting-mimicking diet and then identify how the tumor cell is rewired and how it survives under fasting conditions (see "Fasting and Starvation Escape Routes: The Wild-Card Effect" in chapter 4). This is what we do routinely in our labs at IFOM and USC and what we are starting to test in clinical studies. Soon we hope these starvation escape pathways will be identified rapidly in patients so a low toxicity combination therapy can be selected in a few days and changed later if necessary.

NUTRITION AND KIDNEY CANCER: CLINICAL STUDIES

Ketogenic Diet

There is an ongoing small clinical trial investigating whether the ketogenic diet is safe when combined with the standard of care in patients with metastatic kidney cancer.

In 2021, a French study followed twenty metastatic kidney cancer patients following a 2:1 ketogenic diet (made up of two grams of fat for each gram of protein and carbohydrates) and taking vitamin supplements for one year. The research, still ongoing at the time of publication, is investigating patients' tolerance of the diet and the frequency of adverse events, as well as rates of compliance, progression-free survival, and overall survival after two years.[6]

In order to understand the potential role of a ketogenic diet for kidney cancer in addition to standard treatment, we will need to wait for the results of this study and other larger clinical studies.

KIDNEY CANCER TREATMENT SUMMARY

- Follow standard cancer therapy (chemotherapy, etc.).
- Talk to your oncologist about combining standard therapy with a fasting-mimicking diet, especially in advanced-stage cancers with poor prognosis.
- If this is not sufficient, talk to an oncologist and a dietitian who can help combine a fasting-mimicking diet with a ketogenic diet (low in protein and plant-and-fish-based), making sure it does not negatively affect body mass or immunity function.
- Between treatments, follow the Longevity Diet (see chapter 3).
- Fast for fourteen hours a day (for example, eating only between 8:00 a.m. and 6:00 p.m.) during therapy.
- Maintain a normal body weight.
- Be physically active and exercise, after consulting an oncologist.
- Try to keep your phase angle (an indicator of muscular function) above 5 by doing muscle strength training at least three or four times a week for thirty to forty minutes;

you can follow the exercise video on the Create Cures website's section "Exercise and Longevity."

Patients who would like to learn more about the fasting/nutrition-based interventions described in this chapter should contact the Longevity and Healthspan Clinic of the Create Cures Foundation.

CONCLUSION

This was a particularly difficult book to write for several reasons: on the one hand, it was important to maintain scientific and clinical standards, and on the other hand, I wanted to provide patients with information on the integrative-medicine approach that the oncological community is just starting to pay attention to. This is why I included so many oncologists, doctors, and scientists from some of the leading American and European cancer centers—all of whom have played a key role in contributing their expertise and helping me control my optimism on many occasions, given that there is still a long way to go before we fully understand the effects of the fasting-mimicking diet and of the Longevity Diet in oncology.

My hope is that I, along with my colleagues, will be able to stir up enthusiasm in patients, people at risk, and readers interested in living a long and healthy life by describing the remarkable effect of fasting-mimicking diet cycles against so many cancers in mice and the highly promising initial results from clinical studies combining the fasting-mimicking diet with a variety of cancer drugs.

Personally, I am confident that the fasting-mimicking diet will play an important role in the treatment of various types of cancer in the future. My thoughts on how the system should change have been well established throughout this book, and I hope it helps cancer treatment move in a more patient-focused direction, and does so sooner rather than later, especially for patients with advanced-stage disease and few options. I hope that cancer patients will soon be able to take advantage of a system that is much more sophisticated, fast, and effective than the current one and that will involve both targeted, FDA-approved therapies and wild-card therapies such as the fasting-mimicking diet, implemented by multidisciplinary teams that can take advantage of all the tools available to achieve cures.

APPENDIX 1

Malnutrition Screening and Assessment in Patients with Cancer (for Health-Care Professionals)

Written by Alessandro Laviano, associate professor of medicine in the Department of Translational and Precision Medicine at Sapienza University of Rome

Cancer is considered a systemic and complex disease and requires multiprofessional and multidisciplinary management. Paraneoplastic syndromes—a diffuse set of signs and symptoms triggered by the tumor beyond the affected organ—are frequently diagnosed in patients with advanced disease. Among them, malnutrition is clinically relevant because of its high prevalence and severe impact on patients' outcomes.

As defined by the European Society for Clinical Nutrition and Metabolism (ESPEN), malnutrition is "a state resulting from lack of intake or uptake of nutrition that leads to altered body composition (decreased fat free mass) and body cell mass leading to diminished physical and mental function and impaired clinical outcome from disease." It can be brought on by starvation, disease, or advanced aging, alone or in combination. Cancer-associated malnutrition, also called cachexia, is considered disease-related malnutrition with inflammation, since the inflammatory response induced by the tumor plays a major role in the patient's declining function.

Cachexia, when compared with simple starvation, is a progressive disease characterized by quantitative and qualitative changes of muscle mass with or without wasting of adipose (fat) tissue. Cachexia has a profound influence on clinical outcomes, since it reduces tolerance to anticancer therapies, may cause patients to skip therapy cycles, and impinges on quality of life. Consequently, cancer patients who have cachexia show reduced overall survival. International scientific societies, including ESPEN and the European Society of Medical Oncology (ESMO), consistently recommend nutritional care alongside the treatment of cancer. In particular, patients should be screened for the risk of malnutrition and, if they test positive, should be further assessed.

MALNUTRITION SCREENING TOOLS IN PATIENTS WITH CANCER

The purpose of nutritional screening is to decide whether the patient should receive nutritional treatment (such as supplementation). In general, screening is a quick and simple process that can be conducted by hospital admitting staff or community health-care teams. Nutrition screening tools are designed to detect protein and energy undernutrition, and/or to predict whether undernutrition is likely to develop or worsen. International guidelines recommend the use of the Malnutrition Universal Screening Tool (MUST) or the Nutrition Risk Screening 2002 (NRS-2002), followed by the Short Nutritional Assessment Questionnaire (SNAQ) and the Malnutrition Screening Tool (MST).

- **MUST:** This simple nutrition screening tool was developed by the British Association of Parenteral and Enteral Nutrition. It scores the patient's body mass index (BMI), the degree of weight loss in the previous three to six months, and the acute effects of the disease. When the cumulative score is 2 or greater, the patient could have a high nutritional risk, deserving further assessment and nutritional care.

- **NRS-2002:** This two-step nutrition screening tool initially assesses the clinical features of the patient, including their BMI, the extent of weight loss, current food intake, and severity of disease. If any one of these prompts concern, the screening continues to the second stage, which further explores and scores the severity of the impaired nutritional status and the severity of the underlying disease. A final score of 3 or greater identifies the patient as being at nutritional risk.

- **SNAQ:** This screening tool scores three simple questions: "Did you lose weight unintentionally?" "Did you experience a decreased appetite over the last month?" and "Did you use supplemental drinks or tube feeding over the last month?" A final score of 2 or greater identifies the patient as being at risk, and nutritional care is recommended.

- **MST:** This screening tool considers the presence and severity of unintentional weight loss in the previous months, as well as reduced appetite. A score of 2 or greater identifies the patient as being at risk, and nutritional care is recommended.

MALNUTRITION ASSESSMENT IN PATIENTS WITH CANCER

Cancer-associated malnutrition is a frequent comorbidity, yet it is a risk that can be mitigated.

The best procedure to diagnose malnutrition in cancer patients is still a matter of debate. Since the key features of neoplastic (cancer) cachexia are the quantitative and qualitative changes in muscle mass, the use of imaging techniques seems necessary to diagnose cancer-associated malnutrition. Reliable information on cancer patients' body composition is conveyed by a computed tomography (CT) scan at the level of the third lumbar vertebra. This technique is generally considered the gold standard for measuring muscle mass. However, their cost and the radiation exposure involved make CT scans less feasible to determine whether a patient may be malnourished.[1]

An alternative is nuclear magnetic resonance, but its use is also limited by the high associated cost. Dual-energy X-ray absorptiometry (DEXA) is more affordable but has some radiation risk factors. Another more affordable and safer technique is bioimpedance analysis (BIA), but this is not recommended by international guidelines, since it does not measure muscle mass but derives an estimation of muscle mass from the body's water content. Nevertheless, BIA, as well as the more advanced bioelectrical impedance vector analysis (BIVA), may offer clinically relevant information and can be used when it is not possible to obtain a CT or DEXA scan.

In a large study enrolling 1,139 patients with colorectal cancer undergoing surgery, over half showed reduced muscle mass (sarcopenia) or myosteatosis (fat infiltration in muscle), indicating that for a number of cancers, muscle loss remains a problem to be addressed.

To address the practical challenges of imaging techniques, several alternative approaches have been developed. Handgrip strength is a standardized technique measuring muscle function in the nondominant arm, which has been shown to help predict muscle mass loss in patients with lung cancer receiving nutritional interventions.[2]

By combining BMI and weight-loss amounts, reliable information on patients' survival can be derived. In particular, the worst prognosis is associated with low BMI / high weight loss, whereas the better outcome is associated with high BMI / low weight loss.[3]

More recently, the major international societies of clinical nutrition agreed on a simple procedure to diagnose malnutrition, which can also be used for cancer cachexia. The Global Leadership Initiative on Malnutrition (GLIM) criteria require that after a positive malnutrition screening test by a validated tool, phenotypical (weight loss, low BMI, or reduced muscle mass) and etiologic (reduced food intake or assimilation, inflammation) factors are assessed. The simultaneous presence of a positive nutrition screening and at least one etiologic and one phenotypical factor confirm the diagnosis of malnutrition. (This procedure has recently been endorsed by the ESMO guidelines on cancer cachexia.)

CLINICAL RELEVANCE OF ASSESSING MALNUTRITION IN PATIENTS WITH CANCER

Dependable criteria, however, are still lacking to diagnose cancer-associated malnutrition across countries and centers with varying expertise of personnel and economic resources. Nevertheless, the precise profiling of the nutritional status of patients with cancer can help with the personalization of anticancer therapies, which should include concurrent disease-fighting treatments and symptom-relieving palliative care.

The timely diagnosis of malnutrition helps predict the efficacy and toxicity of anticancer therapies and therefore is a marker for possible tweaks in the therapy to best suit the patient and enhance their quality of life; it also may reduce the costs associated with general management of the disease.

APPENDIX 2

Fasting and Fasting-Mimicking Diet Clinical Studies During Cancer Treatment

Below are summaries of published and ongoing clinical trials, mentioned throughout the book, studying the effects of fasting on cancer treatment, as well as such studies for the prevention of cancer (and other diseases).

The published clinical trials conducted (many in collaboration with my group) include over three thousand patients, with more than six hundred fasting or receiving fasting-mimicking diets (the rest were in the control-diet groups) (see table 1). Overall, the studies suggest that fasting-mimicking diets have proven to be safe and well tolerated in combination primarily with chemotherapy and radiation treatments and have contributed to reducing some adverse effects.

The first study, published in 2009, recorded data on ten patients (four with breast cancer, two with prostate cancer, and one each with ovarian, uterine, non-small-cell carcinoma of the lung, and esophageal adenocarcinoma) who voluntarily chose to fast in conjunction with chemotherapy.

The second study, published in 2015 by Leiden University in the Netherlands, examined the feasibility of short-term fasting and its effects on the tolerance of chemotherapy in a homogeneous group of thirteen patients (of whom seven fasted) with breast or ovarian cancer.

In 2016, we published a clinical trial in which twenty patients followed a water fast for twenty-four, forty-eight, or seventy-two hours in combination with a platinum-based chemotherapy. Taken together, the data from this study showed that seventy-two hours of fasting in combination with chemotherapy is safe and feasible for breast, ovarian, uterine, and lung cancer patients. It also showed a trend of reduced side effects in patients who fasted for seventy-two hours compared with those who fasted for twenty-four hours.

A recent article published in 2018 by researchers from the Charité hospital in Berlin showed that, for patients with gynecological cancer, a fasting-mimicking diet combined with chemotherapy is well tolerated and is associated with an improved quality of life and less fatigue compared with patients receiving a normal diet.

In 2020, a Dutch group of cancer centers published a new study (DIRECT trial) conducted on 131 breast cancer patients, of whom 65 received a fasting-mimicking diet. Here, the breast cancer patients enrolled in the study had HER2-negative tumors. The patients taking part in the study were at stage II/III, indicating a cancer that has grown and may or may not have spread to the surrounding tissues and/or lymph nodes. Patients in the fasting-mimicking-diet group displayed increased clinical response (effect of chemo on tumor size) but also improved pathological response (effect of chemo on the number of active cancer cells within a tumor).

In 2020, we published the results from two clinical trials that included thirty-six patients with hormone receptor positive breast cancer receiving estrogen therapy in combination with cycles of the fasting-mimicking diet. As observed in mice, fasting-mimicking diet cycles caused a reduction in the following factors: insulin (produced by the pancreas when glucose levels in the blood increase), leptin (a hormone produced by fat tissue), and IGF-1 (insulin-like growth factor, which promotes cell—even cancer cell—proliferation). These reductions are of clinical significance because these three factors are associated with cancer growth, so their reduction may negatively affect cancer survival and growth.

In 2021, the same breast cancer patients enrolled in the DIRECT study (described above) were assessed on their quality of life. Specific questionnaires were used to reveal the outcomes at baseline, halfway through chemotherapy, before the last cycle of chemotherapy, and six months after surgery. From the results, the fasting-mimicking diet as an adjunct to neoadjuvant chemotherapy appears to improve certain quality-of-life and illness-perception domains in patients with HER2-negative breast cancer. Even if early clinical studies indicated (table 1) that patients might benefit from regimens of modified fasting, some concerns remained over possible negative impact on the patients' nutritional status. For this reason, this trial assessed the feasibility and safety of the five-day fasting-mimicking diet as well as its effects on body composition and circulating growth factors, adipokines, and cyto/chemokines in ninety cancer patients undergoing active medical treatment. Periodic fasting-mimicking-diet cycles resulted in reduced fat mass, insulin production, and circulating IGF-1 and leptin and were shown to be feasible and safely combined with standard antineoplastic treatments in cancer patients at low nutritional risk.

At the beginning of 2022, a clinical trial involving 101 patients was conducted at the National Cancer Institute in Milan, and its results were published in the journal *Cancer Discovery*. In addition to confirming the metabolic changes that mediate fasting's anticancer effects in preclinical experiments (specifically the safety, feasibility, and consistent reduction of blood glucose and growth-factor concentration associated with the fasting-mimicking diet), this new study revealed a profound reshaping of anticancer immunity through the fasting-mimicking diet. This reshaping led to an improved immunological response to cancer, subsequently associated with better clinical outcomes in a number of cancer patients.

Out of the 101 patients enrolled in the clinical trial above, the researchers reported five cases with exceptional responses involving patients with advanced, poor-prognosis solid neoplasms: one with extensive-stage small-cell lung cancer, one with metastatic pancreatic adenocarcinoma, one with metastatic colorectal cancer, and two with metastatic triple-negative breast cancer. These patients achieved complete and long-lasting tumor remission when treated with a combination of cyclic fasting-mimicking diet and standard systemic treatments. These outcomes were characterized as "exceptional tumor responses," as examined in a paper published in the *European Journal of Cancer* thereafter.

In a 2020 publication in *BMC Cancer*, the results of a cross-pilot study conducted with twenty-two breast cancer patients, two patients with endometrial cancer, two patients with ovarian cancer, and four patients with cervical cancer showed that a four-day fast during chemotherapy can increase patients' tolerance of the treatments and reduce their toxicity.

A qualitative study of patient experience published in the *Journal of Health Psychology* provided data on the motivations to fast and the experience of fasting among a population of women with breast cancer. Results from the study suggest that the motivation is mainly to reduce the negative side effects of chemotherapy. Interestingly, fasting seems to reduce anxiety among patients, since it is associated with a greater sense of control over their treatment. This study also suggests that patients not supported by their doctors on this nutritional strategy may turn to complementary healthcare practitioners.

Another study with eleven ovarian cancer patients, eight uterine cancer patients, and one cervical cancer patient investigated the feasibility and effect of short-term fasting in patients receiving chemotherapy. The results showed that short-term fasting was safe in combination with chemotherapy, that those who fasted required fewer reductions in the dose of chemotherapy or delays in the scheduled treatment, and that the quality of life of these patients improved over the course of treatment.

Another study reported a single clinical case of a forty-two-year-old woman diagnosed with grade 1 follicular lymphoma (stage IIIA, advanced stage). Her only treatment was a water-only fast for twenty-one days and then a plant-based diet free of refined carbohydrates and of added salt, oil, and sugar. She did not receive any other cancer therapy. In the following years, CT/PET scans showed no signs of the cancer. This result, although it needs to be tested by future randomized clinical studies, is in accordance with animal studies on multiple myeloma, which suggest that fasting alone can be very effective against certain—but not all—blood cancers.

In a study aimed at evaluating weight-loss restrictive diets and fasting practices among cancer survivors of the NutriNet-Santé cohort, as well as related sociodemographic and lifestyle factors in about 2,700 cancer survivors, the analysis of questionnaires completed by these patients revealed that after cancer diagnosis, 3.5 percent of patients added some form of fasting to their standard therapies. Fasting was strongly associated with the opinion that such practice could improve cancer prognosis.

In 2020, a group of German clinicians tested the effect of a combination of a ketogenic diet and water-only fasting in glioblastoma patients. The patients received either radiation and a healthy diet or radiation plus a single cycle of six days of a ketogenic diet combined with three days of water-only fasting. This single nine-day dietary change was found to be safe but did not make a significant difference in the glioblastoma progression. After six months, 20 percent of patients on the fasting / ketogenic diet combined with radiation had not progressed, versus 16 percent of those receiving radiation only. As mentioned earlier, a single cycle of fasting is not expected to be effective, based on animal data. Also, the timing of the fasting/fasting-mimicking diet in relation to the therapy is key.

Since the previous study did not meet its primary end point of improved progression-free survival in comparison with a normal diet, the researchers reported their analysis of the diet diaries and the metabolic parameters in a follow-up publication in 2022. The conclusion was that the strict caloric goals of the trial were tolerated well by patients with recurrent brain cancer. The short diet schedule led to significant metabolic changes, with low glucose emerging as a candidate marker of better prognosis, even if the interpretation of the results was complicated by an unexpected lower calorie intake of the control group.

In order to examine the feasibility, safety, systemic biological activity, and cerebral activity of a ketogenic dietary intervention in patients with glioma, twenty-five patients with astrocytoma with stable disease after adjuvant chemotherapy were enrolled in an eight-week nutritional intervention consisting of two fasting days between five modified Atkins diet days (net carbohydrates of no more than twenty grams per day) each week. According to the authors of the study, the dietary intervention, while demanding, produced meaningful cerebral ketone concentration and appears to be a better indicator of systemic activity than patient-reported food records.

There are also several additional ongoing and completed clinical trials studying the effects of fasting diets on the safety and side effects of anticancer therapies, outlined in table 2 below, specifically in breast cancer, melanoma, prostate cancer (including advanced and metastatic), and other solid or hematological tumors. When they are finished, we will have a total of more than eight hundred patient results to bolster the evidence and help us to introduce the fasting-mimicking diet in therapies for some (if not many) cancers. Notably, several of these studies have already been completed, and they both confirm that fasting-mimicking diets are safe and provide initial evidence of efficacy against a variety of cancers in combination with many different therapies.

Overall, these results, even if not yet conclusive, along with the extensive laboratory studies, provide initial evidence for the efficacy and potential of fasting-mimicking diets and should help inspire larger clinical studies to help reduce side effects and improve the effectiveness of a variety of cancer drugs.

To follow up on their findings, you can look for more information at clinicaltrials.gov, a database of privately and publicly funded clinical studies conducted around the world. You'll need the NCT number of the clinical trial (listed in the right-hand column of the tables) to do so.

FEASIBILITY AND SAFETY OF FASTING AND FASTING-MIMICKING DIET FOR PREVENTION OF CANCER (AND OTHER DISEASES)

In 2017, fasting-mimicking diets were tested in healthy adults, including those with risk factors for age-related disease, including high cholesterol, glucose, inflammation, etc. The first study involved one hundred patients in total, and among them, seventy-one received three cycles of a fasting-mimicking diet. The main results pertain to the reduction of blood glucose, IGF-1 (the insulin-like growth factor that promotes cell—even cancer cell—proliferation), body weight, fat, C-reactive protein (an inflammation marker), blood pressure, triglycerides, and cholesterol.[1] These reductions were more noticeable in patients for whom these markers were above the optimal range, suggesting that a fasting-mimicking diet can be a powerful tool in reducing the risk factors for chronic diseases such as cardiovascular, autoimmune, and inflammatory diseases, diabetes, and cancer. A follow-up study of comparable size is yet to be published (at the time of this book's publication) but has confirmed these results. There are now at least four additional trials on patients with hypertension, diabetes, or kidney disease confirming the results above.

TABLE 1: PUBLISHED CLINICAL STUDIES AND REPORTS

	TYPE OF CANCER	PUBLICATION DATE	LOCATION	TYPE OF STUDY	
1	Four patients with breast cancer, two with prostate cancer, and one each with ovarian, uterine, non-small-cell carcinoma of the lung, and esophageal adenocarcinoma	2009	University of Southern California (USC), Los Angeles, United States	Case series report	
2	Breast cancer	2015	Leiden University Medical Center, Netherlands	Randomized pilot study	
3	Six patients with urothelial, six with ovarian, five with breast, two with uterine, one with non-small-cell lung cancer	2016	USC, in collaboration with Norris Comprehensive Cancer Center and the Los Angeles County / USC Medical Center (LAC + USC)	Randomized clinical trial; parallel assignment	
4	Thirty patients with breast and four with ovarian cancer	2018	Charité, Berlin, Germany	Individually randomized crossover trial	
5	Lymphoma	2018	TrueNorth Health Center, Santa Rosa, California, United States	Clinical case	
6	The main cancer locations were prostate, breast, and colorectal	2018	NutriNet-Santé, France	Ongoing web-based cohort study	
7	Breast cancer	2019	Institut du Cancer de Montpellier, France	Qualitative study	
8	Eleven patients with ovarian, eight with uterine, and one with cervical cancer	2020	Graduate School of Medicine, University of Tennessee, Knoxville, United States	Randomized, controlled study	
9	Breast cancer	2020	Leiden University Medical Center in collaboration with Borstkanker Onderzoek Groep and Pink Ribbon, Amsterdam, Netherlands	Multicenter, open-label, randomized DIRECT clinical study	

TABLE 1: PUBLISHED CLINICAL STUDIES AND REPORTS

INTERVENTION	NUMBER OF PATIENTS	NUMBER OF PATIENTS WHO FASTED	NCT NUMBER AND REFERENCE
48–140 hours of fasting prior to and/or following 5–56 hours of chemotherapy	10	10	NCT not available[2]
24 hours before and 24 hours after chemotherapy	13	7	NCT01304251[3]
Water fast 24 or 48 hours before platinum-based chemotherapy or 72 hours (48 pre-chemo and 24 post-chemo)	20	20	NCT00936364[4]
60 hours (36 hours before and 24 hours after chemotherapy)	50	34	NCT01954836[5]
21-day water fast	1	1	NCT not available[6]
Fasting before and after diagnosis, both with and without chemotherapy treatment	2,741	164	NCT03335644[7]
The fast duration ranges from 36 hours and 7 days, started at least 24 hours before chemotherapy	151	16	NCT not available[8]
Fasting 24 hours before and 24 hours after the chemotherapy cycle	20	20	NCT not available[9]
Short-term fasting using fasting-mimicking diet with neoadjuvant chemotherapy	131	65	NCT02126449[10]

TABLE 1: PUBLISHED CLINICAL STUDIES AND REPORTS

	TYPE OF CANCER	PUBLICATION DATE	LOCATION	TYPE OF STUDY	
10	Breast cancer	2020	University of Genoa and Fondazione IRCCS Istituto Nazionale dei Tumori, Milan, Italy	Single-arm, prospective phase II clinical study	
11	Twenty-two patients with breast, four with cervical, two with endometrial and two with ovarian cancer	2020	Department of Oncology and Gynecological Oncology of the Medical Center of the University of Freiburg, Germany	Controlled crossover pilot study	
12	Glioma	2020	Institute of Neurooncology, Frankfurt, and University of Tübingen, Germany	Randomized, parallel assignment, open label	
13	The main cancer locations were breast, hematological, colorectal, prostate, and lung cancers	2021	University of Genoa, Italy	Single-arm, prospective phase II clinical study	
14	Glioma	2021	Wake Forest University Health Sciences, Winston-Salem, North Carolina, United States	Single group assignment	
15	The main cancer locations were breast, colorectal, lung, and prostate cancers	2022	Fondazione IRCCS Istituto Nazionale dei Tumori, Milan, Italy	Monocentric, open-label, single-arm, prospective clinical trial	
16	Two with breast cancer, one with colorectal, one with lung, and one with pancreatic cancer	2022	Fondazione IRCCS Istituto Nazionale dei Tumori, Milan, Italy	Monocentric, open-label, single-arm, prospective clinical trial	
17	Glioma	2022	Institute of Neurooncology, Frankfurt, and University of Tübingen, Germany	Randomized, parallel assignment, open label	

TABLE 1: PUBLISHED CLINICAL STUDIES AND REPORTS

INTERVENTION	NUMBER OF PATIENTS	NUMBER OF PATIENTS WHO FASTED	NCT NUMBER AND REFERENCE
Fasting-mimicking diet repeated every 3 or 4 weeks up to a maximum of 8 consecutive cycles	36	36	NCT03595540 & NCT03340935[11]
4 cycles of 96-hour fasting for half of the chemotherapy cycle	30	30	DRKS00011610[12]
Calorie-restricted, ketogenic diet and transient fasting vs. standard nutrition during reirradiation for patients with recurrent glioblastoma: the ERGO2 Study	50	25	NCT01754350[13]
Fasting-mimicking diet repeated every 3 or 4 weeks	90	90	NCT03595540[14]
2 fasting days interleaved between 5 modified Atkins diet days each week	25	25	NCT0228616[15]
Different combinations of fasting-mimicking diet and standard of care	101	101	NCT03340935[16]
Different combinations of fasting and standard of care	5 (out of the 101)	5 (out of the 101)	NCT03340935[17]
Analysis of diet diaries and metabolic parameters of the ERGO2 trial	50	25	NCT01754350[18]

TABLE 2: ONGOING CLINICAL STUDIES

The patient numbers reported are up to date as of April 4, 2024.

TYPE OF CANCER OR CONDITION	CLINICAL TRIAL TITLE	LOCATION	TYPE OF STUDY	
Breast cancer / melanoma	Impact of Dietary Intervention on Tumor Immunity: The DigesT Trial (DigesT)	Fondazione IRCCS Istituto Nazionale dei Tumori, Milan, Italy	Single arm and three cohorts of patients	
Breast and prostate cancer	Controlled Low Calorie Diet in Reducing Side Effects and Increasing Response to Chemotherapy in Patients with Breast or Prostate Cancer	USC Norris Cancer Center and LAC (Los Angeles General Medical Center), United States	Randomized, phase II clinical trial	
Breast cancer	BRCA Main Home Nutritional Intervention—Random Study	University Hospital, Policlinico Paolo Giaccone, Palermo, Italy	Randomized clinical trial	
Advanced metastatic prostate cancer	Fasting and Nutritional Therapy in Patients with Advanced Metastatic Prostate Cancer	Charité University, Berlin, Germany	Randomized clinical trial	

TABLE 2: ONGOING CLINICAL STUDIES

The patient numbers reported are up to date as of April 4, 2024.

INTERVENTION	NUMBER OF PATIENTS	NUMBER OF PATIENTS WHO FASTED	MAIN AIM OF THE STUDY	NCT NUMBER
5 days fasting-mimicking-diet cycle before or after surgical removal of primary tumor (breast) or lymph nodes (breast, melanoma)	100	93	Assessment of the immunological and metabolic changes induced by the fasting-mimicking diet in the preoperative and postoperative setting	NCT03454282
Fasting-mimicking diet: 3 days prior to chemotherapy, during the 12 weeks of chemotherapy, and 1 day after chemotherapy	130	81	Study of whether the fasting-mimicking diet will reduce chemotherapy toxicity and/or enhance efficacy	NCT01802346
Fasting-mimicking diet every 2 months	300	23	Primary outcomes: IGF-1 and other risk factors	NCT03570125
Modified fasting 36 hours before and 24 hours after chemotherapy	60	49	Assessment of combination of fasting and chemotherapy efficacy	NCT02710721

TABLE 2: ONGOING CLINICAL STUDIES

The patient numbers reported are up to date as of April 4, 2024.

TYPE OF CANCER OR CONDITION	CLINICAL TRIAL TITLE	LOCATION	TYPE OF STUDY	
Platinum-based chemotherapy	Short-Term Fasting: Impact on Toxicity	USC Norris Cancer Center and LAC (Los Angeles General Medical Center), United States	Randomized clinical trial	
LKB1-inactive, advanced lung adenocarcinoma	Metformin Plus/Minus Fasting-Mimicking Diet to Target the Metabolic Vulnerabilities of LKB1-Inactive Lung Adenocarcinoma (FAME)	Fondazione IRCCS Istituto Nazionale dei Tumori, Milan, Italy	Single institution, open label, triple arm, noncomparative phase II trial	
Triple-negative breast cancer (TNBC)	Calorie Restriction with or Without Metformin in Triple Negative Breast Cancer (BREAKFAST)	Fondazione IRCCS Istituto Nazionale dei Tumori, Milan, Italy	Randomized, parallel assignment, open label	
Non-small-cell lung cancer	Fasting-Mimicking Diet with Chemo-immunotherapy in Non–Small Cell Lung Cancer (NSCLC)	Indiana University, United States	Randomized, controlled pilot study	

TABLE 2: ONGOING CLINICAL STUDIES

The patient numbers reported are up to date as of April 4, 2024.

INTERVENTION	NUMBER OF PATIENTS	NUMBER OF PATIENTS WHO FASTED	MAIN AIM OF THE STUDY	NCT NUMBER
Short-term fasting before chemotherapy	70	47	Determination of the safety and feasibility of short-term fasting prior to administration of combination chemotherapy with platinum in patients with advanced solid tumor malignancies	NCT00936364
Fasting-mimicking diet in combination with the standard of care	64	64	Assessment of the efficacy of combining standard-of-care platinum-based chemoimmunotherapy with metformin plus/minus fasting-mimicking diet in patients with LKB1-inactive, advanced lung adenocarcinoma	NCT03709147
6 months of standard preoperative anthracycline plus taxane chemotherapy in combination with 8 triweekly cycles of 5-day fasting-mimicking diet (arm A), or the same chemotherapy / fasting-mimicking diet regimen plus daily metformin (arm B)	90	90	Investigation of the antitumor activity of cyclic fasting-mimicking diet, alone or in combination with metformin, in patients with localized TNBC	NCT04248998
Fasting-mimicking diet in combination with the standard of care	12	12	Evaluation of fasting-mimicking diet in patients receiving chemo-immunotherapy for treatment of metastatic non-small-cell lung cancer	NCT03700437

GLOSSARY

ABIRATERONE: A hormonal medicine that inhibits the production of testosterone and therefore blocks cell growth stimulated by the hormone, which in turn helps kill cancer cells. It is used in prostate cancer therapy.

ACUTE LYMPHOBLASTIC LEUKEMIA (ALL): A type of malignant and progressive leukemia, most common in children.

ACUTE MYELOID LEUKEMIA (AML): A type of malignant leukemia, particularly common in adults and the elderly.

ADENOCARCINOMA: A malignant tumor originating in secretory cells of the glands found in different organs.

ADJUVANT CHEMOTHERAPY: A type of chemotherapy administered after surgery, aimed at increasing the chances of healing and reducing the risk of relapse.

ADRENAL GLANDS: Glands located at the upper end of the kidney, responsible for the production of various hormones that carry out various physiological functions.

AEROBIC EXERCISE: Prolonged physical activity of moderate and constant intensity. The term *aerobic* indicates a type of metabolism in which the cells use oxygen and glucose (sugar) to produce energy. Some examples of aerobic activity are walking, running, and cycling.

ALCOHOL DEHYDROGENASE ENZYME (ADH): An enzyme that digests alcohol, present in the liver and stomach.

ALK GENE: A type of gene involved in signaling to cells and in their growth. Mutated forms of the ALK gene and protein can promote the growth of cancer cells.

AMINO ACIDS: Primary components of proteins.

ANAEROBIC EXERCISE: A type of exercise that causes the body to use glycogen (the reserve of carbohydrates that is formed in the liver) instead of oxygen. It is high-intensity but short-burst physical activity, such as weight lifting or high-intensity interval training (HIIT).

ANDROGENS: Hormones that help the development and maintenance of primary male sexual characters (testicles) and of secondary ones (additional reproductive organs, muscles, beard, and hair).

ANEMIA: A condition characterized by an insufficiency of healthy red blood cells to carry oxygen to body tissues in adequate quantities, causing weakness and fatigue.

ANGIOGENESIS: A process by which new blood vessels are generated from existing ones. In the case of tumor angiogenesis, the new blood vessels cause blood to flow to the tumor mass and therefore help promote tumor growth.

ANTIANGIOGENIC: A drug or treatment that counteracts the process of tumor angiogenesis, or the creation of new blood vessels that encourage tumor growth.

ANTINEOPLASTIC DRUGS: Various types of drugs used for the treatment of tumors, i.e., anticancer drugs.

ANTIOXIDANTS: Substances capable of counteracting, slowing, or neutralizing the formation of oxygen free radicals. These are formed by chemical reactions using oxygen molecules (for cell respiration) and can cause damage to molecules and cell structures.

ANTI-PD-1 THERAPY: An immunotherapy that causes the immune system to attack cancer cells.

APOPTOSIS: The method by which the body causes cell death in order to remove abnormal or damaged cells from the body.

ASTROCYTES: Cells that form the tissue that surrounds and protects the other nerve cells of the brain and spinal cord.

ASTROCYTOMA: A tumor of the central nervous system originating in astrocytes.

BEVACIZUMAB: An anticancer drug belonging to the drug class of angiogenesis inhibitors. It prevents the growth of new blood vessels by targeting a protein called VEGF, which plays a role in angiogenesis.

BIOELECTRICAL IMPEDANCE VECTOR ANALYSIS (BIVA): A technique used to estimate body composition (fat mass and lean mass).

BIOIMPEDANCE ANALYSIS (BIA): A method of measurement used to determine body composition (fat mass and lean mass).

BIOMARKER: A biological molecule found in the blood, in other bodily fluids, or in tissues. It can be used to help detect the presence of a disease.

B LYMPHOCYTES (ALSO CALLED B CELLS): White blood cells that fight infections.

BONE MARROW: Soft tissue contained in bone cavities where blood cells that fight infection (red blood cells, white blood cells, platelets, monocytes, lymphocytes, and neutrophils) are formed.

CA 19-9: A protein found on the cell surface of some tumors and, rarely, in normal tissues in the presence of inflammation or other pathologies. It is released into the bloodstream by cancer cells. It can be used as a tumor marker to detect the presence of pancreatic cancer or other types of cancer.

CARBOHYDRATES: Substances contained mainly in plant food that perform a fundamental function as an energy source. Based on their chemical structure, they are classified into "simple" and "complex" carbohydrates.

CARBOPLATIN: A chemotherapy drug used to treat various forms of cancer, including ovarian cancer, lung cancer, head and neck cancer, brain cancer, and neuroblastoma.

CARCINOMA: Cancer of the epithelial tissues, such as the skin and the tissues that cover or line internal organs.

CARCINOSARCOMA: A malignant tumor made up of a mixture of carcinoma (cancer of the epithelial tissues, such as the skin and the tissues that cover internal organs) and sarcoma (cancer of connective tissues, such as bone, fat, and cartilage).

CATALYST: A substance that quickens or promotes a chemical reaction.

CEA (CARCINOEMBRYONIC ANTIGEN): A protein used as a marker, specifically for colorectal cancer.

CENTERS FOR DISEASE CONTROL AND PREVENTION (CDC): A U.S. federal public health agency that deals with disease control and prevention, accidents, and disabilities.

CHEMOTHERAPY: The administration of one or more drugs that target cancer cells by eliminating them, slowing their growth, or hindering their spread to other tissues.

CHOLESTEROL: A fatty substance present in the blood and in all cells of the body, partially introduced by diet and partially produced in the liver. Although cholesterol is needed in the right amount for the production of cell walls, tissues, hormones, vitamin D, and bile acid, an excessive quantity in the blood (hypercholesterolemia) increases the risk of developing heart disease and stroke.

CHRONIC LYMPHOCYTIC LEUKEMIA (CLL): A cancer of the blood and bone marrow with a slow progression, generally accompanied by the onset of few symptoms in the patient, which is defined as "chronic." In CLL, lymphocytes lose the ability to adequately defend the organs from infections.

CISPLATIN (CDDP): A chemotherapy drug used in the treatment of numerous cancers, including ovarian cancer.

COMORBIDITY: Concomitance of two or more diseases in the same individual.

COMPUTED AXIAL TOMOGRAPHY (CAT) OR COMPUTED TOMOGRAPHY (CT): A procedure that uses a computer to take detailed medical images inside the body; used in radiology for diagnostic purposes.

CORTICOSTEROIDS: Synthetic steroid hormones used as anti-inflammatories and immunosuppressants in numerous therapies.

CRIZOTINIB: An anticancer drug used to stop the growth of lung cancer cells. Acts as an inhibitor of kinase by blocking the proteins produced by the ALK and ROS1 genes used for signaling and growing cells.

CYTOTOXIC TREATMENTS: Any treatment with a toxic effect on cells.

DEXA (DUAL-ENERGY X-RAY ABSORPTIOMETRY): A radiographic technique used primarily to determine bone density; it can also help evaluate nutritional status by quantifying the lean and fat mass in various parts of the body.

DEXAMETHASONE: An anti-inflammatory drug used to reduce the side effects of chemotherapy in cancer patients by raising the level of glucose.

DIFFERENTIAL STRESS SENSITIZATION (DSS): The creation of conditions that make cancer cells but not normal cells more vulnerable to treatment.

DOCOSAHEXAENOIC ACID (DHA): It is a semiessential acid, produced minimally by the body, which must therefore be obtained through diet. It may play a role in transforming tumor cells from being resistant to chemotherapy and radiotherapy to being susceptible to it.

DOUBLE-BLIND PILOT STUDY: An initial small-scale (pilot) study in which neither the subject nor the observer is aware of the treatment administered (double-blind).

DOXORUBICIN: An antibiotic widely used for chemotherapy to treat various types of cancer, including breast cancer.

ENZYMES: Proteins that function as catalysts to stimulate and accelerate various chemical reactions in living organisms; fundamental for cellular function.

EPA (EICOSAPENTAENOIC ACID): A type of omega-3 fatty acid. It is found in fatty cold-water fish (such as salmon) and contributes to reducing the risk of heart disease.

EPENDYMAL CELLS: A type of glial cells of the central nervous system that form the inner lining of the cerebral ventricles.

EPENDYMOMA: A brain tumor formed by ependymal cells (cells that make up the inner lining of the cerebral ventricles).

EPIDERMAL GROWTH FACTOR RECEPTOR (EGFR): A gene that regulates cell growth, differentiation, and survival. In cancer cells, EGFR gene mutations can transmit an excessive growth signal.

EPITHELIAL CELLS: Cells that line the organs.

EPITHELIOMA: A skin tumor, benign or malignant, originating from abundant lining cells in the epidermis called keratinocytes.

ESTROGEN: The hormone responsible for secondary female sexual characteristics (such as breasts and pubic and armpit hair growth), for the menstrual cycle, and for maintenance of pregnancy.

EUROPEAN MEDICINES AGENCY (EMA): The agency of the European Union that oversees the evaluation and the supervision of drugs; it is based in Amsterdam.

FASTING BLOOD SUGAR: The blood glucose level detected in a subject who has fasted for at least eight hours.

FASTING-MIMICKING DIET: A food composition that promotes changes in the body equivalent to those caused by water-only fasting. The diet in most cases lasts from four to seven days and can be repeated cyclically in order to obtain various health benefits. In terms of macronutrients, the fasting-mimicking diet is low in protein and sugar and rich in healthy fats.

FAT: Heterogeneous substances insoluble in water, contained in food of both plant and animal origin. They are defined as "essential fats" if they cannot be synthesized by the human body and are assimilated through diet. Fats perform numerous functions, including the production of energy and energy reserve; they are also fundamental components of cell membranes.

FERRITIN: A protein responsible for the storage of iron in cells.

FIBER: Complex carbohydrates that the human body is unable to manage and absorb. They are found mainly in foods of plant origin, such as fruits and vegetables, whole grains, and legumes and play a fundamental role in intestinal motility.

5-FLUOROURACIL (5-FU): One of the most used chemotherapy drugs to treat colorectal and pancreatic cancers.

FLUOROPYRIMIDINE: An anticancer medicine used in the treatment of solid cancers, such as colorectal cancer.

FOLFIRI: A chemotherapy regimen used in the treatment of colorectal cancer in an advanced and metastatic stage.

FOLFIRINOX: A chemotherapy treatment used primarily to treat pancreatic cancer.

FOLFOX: A chemotherapy treatment used to treat colorectal cancer in an advanced and metastatic stage, similar to the FOLFIRI regimen.

FOOD AND DRUG ADMINISTRATION (FDA): A U.S. government agency that is part of the Department of Health and Human Services, responsible for the protection and promotion of public health.

FREE RADICALS: Toxic molecules that can damage DNA and many other cell components and cause cancer cells to commit suicide.

G-CSF (GRANULOCYTE-COLONY STIMULATING FACTOR): A protein that stimulates the growth of white blood cells, which are essential for the protection of the body from infections. Drugs containing G-CSF are used to counteract the reduction of white blood cells in patients undergoing chemotherapy.

GEMCITABINE: A chemotherapy drug used to counter several types of cancer, including ovarian cancer.

GLIAL CELLS: Cells of the nervous system that protect and support the development of neurons.

GLIOBLASTOMA (GLIOBLASTOMA MULTIFORME, GBM): A very aggressive brain tumor, belonging to the category of astrocytoma. It is among the most severe gliomas (brain tumors) because it is characterized by a high growth rate of the tumor mass.

GLIOMA: The most common brain tumor, which starts from the glial cells of the nervous system. There are different types, depending on the cells affected and the rate of tumor growth.

GLUCOCORTICOIDS: A class of steroid hormones, like cortisol and corticosterone, produced by the adrenal cortex; they are involved in glucose metabolism.

GLUCOSE: A simple carbohydrate that is an important energy source for both plant and animal organisms.

GLYCOGEN: A polymer (large, high-weight molecule) of glucose found as a reserve of carbohydrates formed in the liver.

GROWTH HORMONE RECEPTOR (GHR): Protein encoded by the GHR gene that regulates growth signaling and aging, as well as metabolism and various other physiological processes.

GYNECOLOGICAL TUMORS: Tumors affecting the female reproductive systems, especially the uterus and ovaries.

HAYFLICK LIMIT: The capacity threshold of human cells to divide and generate other cells identical to them, which is caused by the shortening of telomeres.

HEMATOCRIT: Percentage of blood volume made up of red blood cells.

HEMATOLOGICAL (OR HEMATOPOIETIC MALIGNANT) TUMORS: Tumors affecting the blood, bone marrow, and lymph nodes, including several types of leukemia.

HEMATURIA: The presence of blood in the urine. It can be traced back to a urinary tract tumor or to other pathologies.

HEMOGLOBIN: A protein found in red blood cells that transports oxygen from the lungs to tissues and organs and returns carbon dioxide to the lungs.

HER2 (HUMAN EPIDERMAL GROWTH FACTOR RECEPTOR 2): A protein that regulates normal cell growth and is found in large quantities in some cancer cells that grow and spread rapidly. A test to check for its presence can help plan treatment, including medications that specifically target this protein.

HER2-NEGATIVE CANCER: A type of carcinoma characterized by HER2-negative cells. These cells have low or no levels of a protein called HER2 (which regulates growth in healthy cells); therefore, they grow more slowly and are less likely to recur or spread to other parts of the body compared with HER2-positive cancer cells.

HORMONE THERAPY: A treatment aimed at adding, removing, or blocking hormones in order to slow the growth of or destroy cancer cells.

HYPERBARIC OXYGEN THERAPY: A therapy consisting of breathing in pure oxygen in a pressurized environment (characterized by pressure levels much higher than atmospheric).

HYPERURICEMIA: An accumulation in the blood of uric acid waste, which is the final product of the metabolism of purines, substances ingested through some foods and drinks as well as produced by the body.

IFOSFAMIDE: A drug used to treat certain testicular cancers and other types of cancer.

IMMUNOTHERAPY: A therapy that uses substances to stimulate or suppress the immune system in order to help the body fight cancer, infections, and other diseases. Some types of immunotherapies are aimed only at certain cells of the immune system, while others act on the immune system in general.

IMMUNOTHERAPY DRUGS: Drugs that stimulate or suppress the immune system to help the body fight cancer.

INHIBITOR: A substance that slows down or stops a chemical reaction. It is used to block cellular signaling pathways.

INSULIN: A hormone that lowers blood glucose levels; produced by the beta cells of the pancreas.

INSULIN-LIKE GROWTH FACTOR 1 (IGF-1): A factor that promotes cell growth and survival. It contributes to aging and tumors.

INTERMITTENT FASTING: A practice that involves abstaining from food for a period ranging from twelve to twenty-four hours daily or every other day

INTERNATIONAL AGENCY FOR RESEARCH ON CANCER (IARC): An international organization that conducts and coordinates research on the causes of cancer and collects data on the incidence of cancer all over the world.

INTESTINAL MICROBIOTA (ALSO CALLED INTESTINAL FLORA, GUT MICROBIOTA, OR GUT FLORA): A population of bacteria and other microorganisms present in the intestine.

IRON: A mineral that the body needs to produce hemoglobin. It is found in red meat, fish, lentils, beans, and grains.

JUVENTOLOGY: The study of youth and the "health interval" (health span), i.e., the period of life during which a person remains young and healthy.

KERATINOCYTES: The main cells that make up the skin, constituting about 95 percent of the organ.

KETOGENESIS: An increase in ketone bodies.

KETOGENIC DIET: A diet with normal calorie intake, rich in fat and low in carbohydrates (the classic proportion between the macronutrients is four parts fat to one part carbohydrates and proteins), which causes the body to break down fat into molecules called ketone bodies.

KETONE BODIES: Chemicals produced when lipids are used as an energy source in place of glucose, when the latter is not present in sufficient quantities in the body.

KETOSIS: When an organism uses fats and ketone bodies to get energy.

KINASE: A type of enzyme (protein that accelerates chemical reactions in the body) capable of regulating numerous cellular processes, especially the transmission of signals inside the cell. It works by modifying sugars or proteins by adding phosphates (molecules composed of phosphorus and oxygen) in a process called phosphorylation.

KINASE INHIBITORS: Small molecules that target certain growth genes that are activated in certain types of cancer. They block kinase and the growth of new blood vessels that tumors need to grow. Examples are rapamycin, crizotinib, and sorafenib.

KRAS GENE MUTATIONS: Genetic mutations among the most commonly linked to cancer; they are common in lung, pancreatic, and colorectal cancer and can metastasize. In healthy cells, the KRAS gene works as an on-off switch that regulates cell growth, but if changed, it can remain stuck in the "on" position, leading to the uncontrolled cell growth.

LARON SYNDROME: A condition characterized by a deficiency of growth hormone receptors and low levels of insulin-like growth factor 1 (IGF-1), which leads those affected to have a smaller stature.

LEPTIN: A protein produced by fat cells that plays a role in the regulation of appetite and fat storage.

LEUCOVORIN: A derivative of folic acid (vitamin B9) used to counteract folic acid deficiency.

LEUKEMIA: A cancer of the blood caused by the production of abnormal blood cells, originating from the tissues that create the blood (such as bone marrow).

LONGEVITY DIET: A diet that aims to slow down cellular aging and reduce the risk of the onset of cardiovascular and autoimmune diseases, diabetes, and neurodegenerative diseases such as Alzheimer's. It is a vegan diet with the addition of fish two or three times a week, where legumes are the main source of protein. Fats and sugars are reduced to a minimum, but the diet includes complex carbohydrates, olive oil, and nuts. It is recommended to eat within an eleven- to twelve-hour span and fast for twelve to thirteen hours a day.

LYMPHATIC SYSTEM: A set of tissues and organs (including the bone marrow, spleen, thymus, and lymph nodes) that produce and store the cells that fight infections and diseases.

LYMPHEDEMA: A condition in which excess fluid collects in the tissues and causes swelling, although it is usually painless. It occurs due to removal of or damage to the lymph nodes caused by cancer treatment.

LYMPH NODES: Small glands that are part of the lymphatic system and have a fundamental role in immunity, trapping bacteria and cancer cells that travel through the body via the lymphatic fluid.

LYMPHOCYTES: A type of white blood cells responsible for immune responses. The two main types of lymphocytes are B cells, which produce antibodies that attack bacteria and toxins, and T cells, which attack other cells when they are attacked by viruses or have become cancerous.

LYMPHOMA: A cancer of the blood originating from the lymphocytes of the immune system.

MAGNESIUM: A metal and an essential nutrient for all cell types, involved in many body processes including nerve signaling, the development of healthy bones, and normal muscle contraction.

MAGNETIC RESONANCE IMAGING (MRI): A technique used for the diagnosis of various illnesses. It generates detailed images of the human body using magnetic fields, avoiding surgery or radiation.

MELANOCYTES: Cells in the skin and the eyes that make and contain melanin; they're found in the epidermis, hair bulb, ocular uveal membrane, pigment epithelium of the retina, and iris.

MELANOMA: A malignant skin tumor that develops from melanocytes, the cells that produce the pigment called melanin; it often comes in the form of a mole. It is among the most dangerous of skin cancers.

MESOTHELIOMA: A malignant tumor of the mesothelium (the lining of the cavities of the body and its organs). It occurs most commonly in the thoracic cavity

METABOLIC PATHWAYS: An ordered and linked series of chemical reactions catalyzed by enzymes in the cell.

METABOLISM: A set of biochemical reactions necessary for maintaining, renewing, and growing cells and organisms.

METASTASIS: Cancer cells that have spread from their originating organ to other parts of the body.

METHYLPREDNISOLONE: A synthetic glucocorticoid with anti-inflammatory, immunosuppressive, and antiallergic properties.

MICROBIOTA: A population of microorganisms that live in the human body without damaging it. The intestinal microbiota is made up of microorganisms belonging to the intestine.

MINERALS: Micronutrients used by the body to regulate body fluids and the vital processes of cells, for the formation of bones, and in many metabolic processes. Calcium, phosphorus, and magnesium are all minerals, along with potassium, chlorine, sodium, and iron.

MINIMALLY INVASIVE SURGERY: A treatment designed as an alternative to radical operations.

MITOCHONDRIA: Organelles (specialized structures within most cells) in which most of the energy needed for cells' biochemical reactions is produced.

MULTICENTER STUDY: A study carried out in several locations (such as hospitals or universities) using the same protocol; all the data is processed by a single coordinator who analyzes the results.

MYELOMA: A cancer that affects white blood cells, essential for the production of antibodies.

MYOSTEATOSIS: An infiltration or accumulation of fat in the muscles.

NEOADJUVANT CHEMOTHERAPY: Chemotherapy administered prior to surgery, aimed at optimizing the result of surgical treatment.

NEOPLASIA: Abnormal cell growth, which may be benign or malignant.

NEOPLASTIC CACHEXIA: Tumor-related malnutrition, characterized by quantitative and qualitative changes in muscle mass, with or without loss of adipose (fat) tissue.

NEOPLASTIC CELLS: Cells that multiply abnormally compared with other cells in the same area of the body, creating damage to the organism. Synonymous with the term *cancer cells*.

NEOPLASTIC DISEASE: A condition that causes the development of tumors, either malignant or benign.

NEULASTA: A drug that stimulates the growth of white blood cells and reduces the risk of infections.

NEUROBLASTOMA: A tumor originating from cells of the nervous system; most common in infants and children. It is formed from the neuroblasts (mature or developing nerve cells present in the sympathetic nervous system that control involuntary bodily functions such as the heartbeat) and spreads throughout the body. It usually begins in the adrenal glands, but it can also begin in the abdomen, the chest, or nerve tissue near the spine.

NEUROPATHY: Nerve disease or malfunction.

NEUTROPENIA: An abnormally low number of neutrophils.

NEUTROPHILS: A type of white blood cells belonging to the category of granulocytes, which have small sacs (granules) containing enzymes that digest microorganisms. Also known as polymorphonuclear leukocytes.

NON-HODGKIN'S LYMPHOMAS (NHL): A heterogeneous group of malignant tumors that originate from B and T lymphocytes. They differ from Hodgkin's lymphomas because of the absence of a particular type of cancer cells.

NON-SMALL-CELL LUNG CANCER (NSCLC): A type of lung cancer that has larger cancer cells than small-cell lung cancer. Also known as nonmicrocitoma.

NUTRITECHNOLOGY: A set of cutting-edge technologies and analytical methods based on traditional human nutrition research.

OLIGODENDROCYTES: Cells in the glia that produce myelin, a substance that coats and protects nerve fibers.

OLIGODENDROGLIOMA: A rare brain tumor of the glia that originates in oligodendrocytes and occurs mainly in the cortex and white matter of the cerebral hemispheres.

OMEGA-3: Essential fatty acids that lower the level of LDL ("bad") cholesterol in the blood. They are found in fish oils and some plant-based foods and are used to combat high triglycerides, rheumatoid arthritis, depression, some forms of dementia, and asthma.

ONCOGENES: Mutated genes that have the potential to cause cancer. These are transformed versions of the same genes that promote normal cell growth and that accelerate aging (e.g., RAS, AKT, PKA).

OSTEOPOROSIS: A condition characterized by the loss of bone mass and density, which causes brittle bones and fractures.

OXALIPLATIN: A chemotherapy drug that binds to DNA and interferes with the stages of the cell cycle, causing the death of cancer cells. It is used to treat advanced-stage cancers, including colorectal cancer.

PALBOCICLIB: A drug used to treat breast cancer and prevent its growth.

PALLIATIVE CARE (ALSO CALLED SUPPORTIVE CARE): Treatment aimed at preventing or treating the side effects (pain and other symptoms) caused by a specific treatment. It is often administered after the primary therapeutic treatment with the aim of increasing the patient's tolerance of therapies and mitigating physical deterioration, so as to improve the patient's quality of life. It is often misidentified as care administered during the terminal phase of the disease.

PARANEOPLASTIC SYNDROME: Symptoms beyond the effects on the affected organ, often diagnosed in patients with advanced cancer. An example is cancer cachexia.

PENICILLIN: An antibiotic used to treat many infections.

PESCATARIAN DIET: A semivegetarian diet that excludes meat from land animals and birds but includes fish, mollusks, and crustaceans, as well as animal derivatives such as dairy products, eggs, and honey, and all foods of plant origin, such as cereals, fruits and vegetables, legumes, seeds, and nuts.

PHASE ANGLE (BIOIMPEDANCE): An indicator of muscle function measured by bioimpedance.

PILOT STUDY: A small-scale preliminary study to evaluate whether a therapy is safe and feasible.

PLATELETS (THROMBOCYTES): Small cells (megakaryocytes) located in the blood and spleen. They assist in the clotting process of the blood.

PLEURAL EFFUSION: An accumulation of fluids between the layers of the pleura, tissue that lines the lungs and chest cavity.

POLYCYTHEMIA: A rare blood cancer caused by an alteration of bone marrow cells that leads to an uncontrolled production of blood cells.

POLYPHENOLS: Substances present in the plant world that give color to some flowers, fruits, and vegetables and have antioxidant properties.

POLYUNSATURATED FATTY ACIDS (PUFA): A type of fatty acids important for the health of cell membranes. An example is the omega-3 fatty acid docosahexaenoic acid (DHA).

POSITRON EMISSION TOMOGRAPHY (PET): A diagnostic technique that involves intravenously administering a radioactive drug; used to detect a disease, such as cancer, or to monitor the effectiveness of a cancer treatment.

PREDNISOLONE: A steroid drug that exerts an anti-inflammatory and immunosuppressive function.

PROBIOTICS: Live microorganisms used as food supplements to help digestion and normal intestinal function. The most common probiotic is *Lactobacillus acidophilus*, found in yogurt.

PROGESTERONE: A hormone released by the ovary with a role in the menstrual cycle and in the early stages of pregnancy.

PROGRAMMED CELL DEATH PROTEIN 1 (PD-1): A protein present on the surface of certain types of immune cells that contributes to controlling the body's immune responses.

PROTEIN: A molecule composed of amino acids. Proteins are the basis of bodily structures, such as skin and hair, and of the most fundamental substances for the body, such as enzymes, cytokines, and antibodies.

PROSPECTIVE STUDY: A study in which patients are monitored from the start of the study to its conclusion. It is different from a retrospective study, which focuses on events prior to the start of the study.

PROTO-ONCOGENE: A gene involved in cell growth. Mutations in a proto-oncogene can make it become an oncogene, which can cause the growth of cancer cells.

PSA (PROSTATE-SPECIFIC ANTIGEN) TEST: A blood test that detects a protein produced by the prostate; used for early detection and control of prostate cancer in asymptomatic patients.

RADICAL PROSTATECTOMY: Surgery that is a partial or total removal of the prostate and part of the surrounding tissue, including the seminal vesicles (glands that help produce sperm).

RADIOTHERAPY: A treatment with high-energy ionizing radiation, often used to kill cancer cells and prevent their growth and multiplication in the area being treated. Radiation can come from a machine (external radiation) or from an implant placed in or near the tumor (internal radiation).

RANDOMIZED CLINICAL TRIAL: A clinical study in which participants are assigned randomly to different groups that either receive the treatment or do not receive the treatment (control group), with the aim of quantifying the effect of the treatment on patients.

RAPAMYCIN: A kinase inhibitor. It inhibits the signaling pathway mTOR-S6K involved in growth, and many other cellular functions.

RAS-PKA: One of the main signaling routes that accelerates aging, activated by glucose or growth factors.

RASVAL19: A yeast genetic mutation similar to a mammal's oncogenic mutation.

REACTIVE OXYGEN MOLECULES: Molecules that promote apoptosis (programmed cell death) by activating processes of cell suicide in tumor cells.

RECEPTORS: Proteins capable of binding to certain hormones. Some cancer cells have hormone receptors and need hormones to grow, while others have no receptors and grow in the absence of these hormones. Knowing if the cancer is hormone receptor positive or negative can help in treatment planning.

RELAPSE-FREE SURVIVAL: A time period after treatment in which the patient survives without signs or symptoms of cancer. Measuring relapse-free survival is a way to evaluate the effectiveness of new treatments.

RENAL CELL CARCINOMA (RCC): One of the two types of kidney cancer that occur in adults. It is the most widespread form and has its origin in the largest part of the kidney (cortex and medulla).

RENAL TRANSITIONAL-CELL CARCINOMA (RTCC): One of the two types of kidney cancer that occur in adults. It forms in the renal pelvis.

REPLICATIVE SENESCENCE: The cell division-dependent decline of cells' capacity to generate new cells, associated with cellular aging.

ROS1 GENE: Gene involved in signaling to cells and in their growth. Mutated forms of the ROS1 gene and protein can promote the growth of cancer cells and have been found in some cancers, including non-small-cell lung cancer (NSCLC), glioblastoma multiforme (a type of brain cancer), and cancers of the bile duct, ovary, stomach, colon, and rectum.

SARCOMA: A type of cancer that starts in the bones or soft tissues of the body, such as cartilage, fat, muscle, blood vessels, fibrous tissues, or other connective or supporting tissues.

SARCOPENIA: A reduction in muscle mass associated with natural aging.

SCH9: The yeast version of the mammalian S6K gene.

SENTINEL LYMPH NODES: The first lymph nodes affected by metastasis. The sentinel lymph node provides information on the possible spread of the tumor.

SHORT-TERM FASTING: The practice of abstaining from food for twelve to forty-eight to seventy-two hours.

SIGNALING ROUTES: Mechanisms for transmitting signals from the outside to the inside of a cell.

SMALL-CELL LUNG CANCER (SCLC): A type of lung cancer named for the small size of its tumor cells observed under the microscope. Also known as microcitoma. It accounts for about 15 to 20 percent of cases of malignant lung tumors.

SODIUM: A mineral abundant in the body that regulates the balance of fluids and is present in the blood and connective tissues, bone tissue, and cartilaginous tissues.

SOLID TUMORS: Tumors formed by a mass with a similar structure to healthy cellular tissue. They are different from blood cancer and lymph cancer, in which cancer cells are suspended in fluids.

SPINAL CORD: The structure belonging to the central nervous system and located inside the vertebral canal. It connects the brain with the rest of the body.

STAGE (OF A TUMOR): The classification of a tumor according to its size, location, and characteristics.

STARCH: A complex carbohydrate found in pasta, rice, potatoes, and some fruits, such as apples, bananas, and mangoes.

SYMPATHETIC NERVOUS SYSTEM: The nervous system activated in conditions of stress and in emergency situations, as opposed to the parasympathetic nervous system, which regulates functions at rest. Both nervous systems control involuntary bodily functions.

TAMOXIFEN: A hormone therapy drug that blocks the action of estrogen in the treatment of breast cancer.

TAXOL: A chemotherapy drug that inhibits cell division.

TELOMERASE: An enzyme activated by cancer cells that is capable of maintaining the telomere long enough for the cell to continue to grow.

TELOMERES: Small segments of DNA at the ends of chromosomes. If they are sufficiently long, the cell can continue to generate new cells. Once the telomeres are shortened, cell growth stops and the cell is called "senescent," or old.

TESTOSTERONE: A hormone produced mainly in the testes necessary to develop and maintain male sexual characteristics. It can also be produced in a laboratory and is used to treat certain medical conditions.

THROMBOCYTOPENIA: A condition characterized by a low number of platelets (thrombocytes), which are important for blood clotting and internal rupture of bleeding.

T LYMPHOCYTES (ALSO CALLED T CELLS): White blood cells that play a central role in fighting infections and cancer.

TOXICITY: The ability of a chemical or pharmaceutical substance to cause damage to living organisms (animals or plants) that ingest it or come into contact with it.

TOXINS: Waste products derived from metabolic pathways (e.g., free radicals from mitochondria) or substances in the external environment (such as from a poor diet or from pollution). They are usually eliminated from the body, but if excessive can be deposited in the tissues.

TRIGLYCERIDES: Fats that enter the body mainly through diet, with a small percentage produced by the liver.

TRIPLE-NEGATIVE BREAST CANCER: A type of breast cancer in which cancer cells have neither estrogen receptors nor progesterone receptors nor large amounts of HER2 protein on their surface.

25-HYDROXYVITAMIN D, OR 25(OH)D: A form of vitamin D that is absorbed and metabolized by the liver and useful for bone growth and health. Monitoring 25-hydroxyvitamin D is essential in patients diagnosed with pathologies such as osteoporosis and rickets.

UROGRAPH: A radiological test that examines the urinary tract, i.e., the organs and ducts through which urine passes.

VASCULAR ENDOTHELIAL GROWTH FACTOR (VEGF): A signaling protein that promotes the growth of new blood vessels (angiogenesis). It contributes to the growth of tumors and is inhibited by some anticancer drugs.

VITAMIN C: A nutrient that the body needs in small quantities to stay healthy. It helps fight infections and heal wounds and aids tissue health.

WARBURG EFFECT: The modification of cellular metabolism in tumor cells to get more energy from sugars and a cellular process called glycolysis, rather than from the mitochondria (which are severely damaged in cancer cells). It was discovered by the German biochemist and physician Otto Warburg.

ACKNOWLEDGMENTS

I would like to offer my thanks to the numerous colleagues and especially the oncologists who have offered me their valuable advice and support during this project—this book would not be the same without their input.

Special thanks go to Professor Alessandro Laviano, whose leadership in the field of oncological nutrition improved the book, especially those parts related to the treatment and prevention of malnutrition in patients.

I thank Gilda Nappo for all the images in this book and the illustrator and artist Manuela Lupis for her work and expertise.

I also offer my thanks to our nutritionists Francesca Valdemarin, Nicole Labaguer, Alessandra Fedato, Alessandro Ciocia, Angelica Nobili, Maura Bozzali, Elisa Pierella, Viviana Dello Ioio, Chiara Nardone, Marta Veneziano, Ghina Al Haj, Giorgia Calori, Silvia Fain, Eleonora Luvarà, and Dr. Ilaria Faggi, as well as our students Francesca Paniccia and Elenora di Luzio for their research of scientific material and constant support in all my foundation's work.

Thanks also to Dr. Giulia Mentrasti for reviewing the manuscript, and to our Bocconi University interns, Giulia Gandino, Ioana Caraghiozov, and Mattia De Carli, for helping with the bibliography; Anita Ciarlo, Giulia Carra, and Ilaria Giabbani for their support in the preparation of the glossary, the translation of the legends of the images, and revision of the bibliography; and Maggie Capodaglio, Achraf Fadhel, Gilda Noschese, and Charlotte Zenatelli for their collaboration on the English edition.

My gratitude goes to the whole Valter Longo Foundation and Create Cures Foundation, but especially to Romina Inés Cervigni and Cristina Villa for their constant support and dedication to this book. Romina and Cristina helped generate a book far better than what I could have written on my own—and on time! I thank Antonluca Matarazzo, executive director of the Create Cures Foundation in Los Angeles and CEO and vice president of the Valter Longo Foundation in Italy. Thanks also to Marco Capace, our social media and digital marketing collaborator, and our collaborator Camilla Colciago Conti for their support in communication and promotion activities. I also thank our collaborators Marco Paonessa, director of strategic initiatives at the Create Cures Foundation in Los Angeles, and Rita Bonzio, head of fundraising, marketing, and communications at the Valter Longo Foundation in Italy.

I thank Kathryn Huck and Hannah Steigmeyer for editing the book.

I thank Laurie Liss at Sterling Lord Literistic for her guidance and support. I also thank the whole Avery team at Penguin Random House.

Special thanks go to AIRC (Italian Association for Cancer Research) for funding our most important cancer research in the 2014–2024 period.

NOTES

INTRODUCTION

1. National Cancer Institute, "Alcohol and Cancer Risk," n.d., viewed July 10, 2023, cancer.gov/about-cancer/causes-prevention/risk/alcohol/alcohol-fact-sheet.
2. American Cancer Society, "Lifetime Risk of Developing or Dying from Cancer," n.d., viewed July 10, 2023, cancer.org/cancer/risk-prevention/understanding-cancer-risk/lifetime-probability-of-developing-or-dying-from-cancer.html.
3. Cancer Research UK, "Lifetime Risk of Cancer," n.d., viewed July 10, 2023, cancerresearchuk.org/health-professional/cancer-statistics/risk/lifetime-risk#heading-Zero.
4. Associazione Italiana di Oncologia Medica, Associazione Italiana Registri Tumori, and Società Italiana di Anatomia Patologica e di Citopatologia Diagnostica, "I numeri del cancro in Italia 2020," n.d., viewed July 10, 2023, aiom.it/wp-content/uploads/2020/10/2020_Numeri_Cancro-operatori_web.pdf.
5. A molecular biologist studies the chemistry of cancer at a molecular level.
6. Maira Di Tano et al., "Synergistic Effect of Fasting-Mimicking Diet and Vitamin C Against KRAS Mutated Cancers," *Nature Communications* 11, no. 1 (May 2020): 2332, DOI:10.1038/s41467-020-16243-3.
7. U.S. Food and Drug Administration, "Expanded Access | Keywords, Definitions, and Resources," n.d., viewed: July 10, 2023, fda.gov/news-events/expanded-access/expanded-access-keywords-definitions-and-resources.

1. FASTING CANCER, FEEDING PATIENTS

1. Douglas Hanahan and Robert A. Weinberg, "Hallmarks of Cancer: The Next Generation," *Cell* 144, no. 5 (2011): 646–74, DOI:10.1016/j.cell.2011.02.013.

2. Stefano Di Biase et al., "Fasting-Mimicking Diet Reduces HO-1 to Promote T Cell–Mediated Tumor Cytotoxicity," *Cancer Cell* 30, no. 1 (July 11, 2016): 136–46, DOI:10.1016/j.ccell.2016.06.005.
3. Di Biase et al., "Fasting-Mimicking Diet Reduces HO-1."
4. Stefano Di Biase et al., "Fasting Regulates EGR1 and Protects from Glucose- and Dexamethasone-Dependent Sensitization to Chemotherapy," *PLOS Biology* 15, no. 3 (March 30, 2017): e2001951, DOI:10.1371/journal.pbio.2001951.
5. Mary Ann Weiser et al., "Relation Between the Duration of Remission and Hyperglycemia During Induction Chemotherapy for Acute Lymphocytic Leukemia with a Hyperfractionated Cyclophosphamide, Vincristine, Doxorubicin, and Dexamethasone/Methotrexate-Cytarabine Regimen," *Cancer* 100, no. 6 (March 15, 2004): 1179–85, DOI:10.1002/cncr.20071.
6. Hanahan and Weinberg, "Hallmarks of Cancer."

2. GENES, AGING, AND CANCER

1. Maggie Vergara et al., "Hormone-Treated Snell Dwarf Mice Regain Fertility but Remain Long Lived and Disease Resistant," *Journal of Gerontology: Series A* 59, no. 12 (2004): 1244–55, DOI:10.1093/gerona/59.12.1244.
2. Yuji Ikeno et al., "Reduced Incidence and Delayed Occurrence of Fatal Neoplastic Diseases in Growth Hormone Receptor/Binding Protein Knockout Mice," *Journal of Gerontology: Series A* 64A, no. 5 (2009): 522–29, DOI:10.1093/gerona/glp017.
3. Andrzej Bartke, Liou Y. Sun, and Valter Longo, "Somatotropic Signaling: Trade-offs Between Growth, Reproductive Development, and Longevity," *Physiological Reviews* 93, no. 2 (2013): 571–98, DOI:10.1152/physrev.00006.2012.
4. Jaime Guevara-Aguirre et al., "Growth Hormone Receptor Deficiency Is Associated with a Major Reduction in Pro-Aging Signaling, Cancer, and Diabetes in Humans," *Science Translational Medicine* 3, no. 7 (2011): 70ra13, DOI:10.1126/scitransl-med.3001845.
5. Zvi Laron et al., "IGF-I Deficiency, Longevity and Cancer Protection of Patients with Laron Syndrome," *Mutation Research: Reviews in Mutation Research* 772 (2017): 123–33, DOI:10.1016/j.mrrev.2016.08.002.
6. Irene Caffa et al., "Fasting-Mimicking Diet and Hormone Therapy Induce Breast Cancer Regression," *Nature* 583, no. 7817 (2020): 620–24, DOI:10.1038/s41586-020-2957-6, author correction in *Nature* 588, no. 7839 (December 2020): E33.

3. FASTING, NUTRITION, AND PHYSICAL ACTIVITY IN CANCER PREVENTION

1. Shubhroz Gill and Satchidananda Panda, "A Smartphone App Reveals Erratic Diurnal Eating Patterns in Humans That Can Be Modulated for Health Benefits," *Cell Metabolism* 22, no. 5 (November 3, 2015): 789–98, DOI:10.1016/j.cmet.2015.09.005.

2. Huashan Bi et al., "Breakfast Skipping and the Risk of Type 2 Diabetes: A Meta-Analysis of Observational Studies," *Public Health Nutrition* 18, no. 16 (November 2015): 3013–19, DOI:10.1017/S1368980015000257.

3. H. M. Bloch , J. R. Thornton, and K. W. Heaton, "Effects of Fasting on the Composition of Gallbladder Bile," *Gut* 21, no. 12 (December 1980): 1087–89, DOI:10.1136/gut.21.12.1087; R. Sichieri, J. E. Everhart, and H. Roth, "A Prospective Study of Hospitalization with Gallstone Disease Among Women: Role of Dietary Factors, Fasting Period, and Dieting," *American Journal of Public Health* 81, no. 7 (July 1991): 880–84, DOI:10.2105/ajph.81.7.880; R. Ofori-Asenso, A. J. Owen, and D. Liew, "Skipping Breakfast and the Risk of Cardiovascular Disease and Death: A Systematic Review of Prospective Cohort Studies in Primary Prevention Settings," *Journal of Cardiovascular Development and Disease* 6, no. 3 (August 2019): 30, DOI:10.3390/jcdd6030030.

4. Gill and Panda, "Smartphone App Reveals."

5. Catherine R. Marinac et al., "Prolonged Nightly Fasting and Breast Cancer Prognosis," *JAMA Oncology* 2, no. 8 (August 1, 2016): 1049–55, DOI:10.1001/jamaoncol.2016.0164.

6. Min Wei et al., "Fasting-Mimicking Diet and Markers/Risk Factors for Aging, Diabetes, Cancer, and Cardiovascular Disease," *Science Translational Medicine* 9, no. 377 (2017): eaai8700, DOI:10.1126/scitranslmed.aai8700; Irene Caffa et al., "Fasting-Mimicking Diet and Hormone Therapy Induce Breast Cancer Regression," *Nature* 583, no. 7817 (2020): 620–24, DOI:10.1038/s41586-020-2502-7, author correction in *Nature* 588 (December 2020): E33, DOI:10.1038/s41586-020-2957-6.

7. Ricki J. Colman et al., "Caloric Restriction Delays Disease Onset and Mortality in Rhesus Monkeys," *Science* 325, no. 5937 (2009): 201–4, DOI:10.1126/science.1173635; Ricki J. Colman et al., "Caloric Restriction Reduces Age-Related and All-Cause Mortality in Rhesus Monkeys," *Nature Communications* 5 (April 1, 2014): 3557, DOI:10.1038/ncomms4557; Julie A. Mattison et al., "Impact of Caloric Restriction on Health and Survival in Rhesus Monkeys from the NIA Study," *Nature* 489, no. 7415 (2012): 318–21, DOI:10.1038/nature11432.

8. Junya Kanda et al., "Impact of Alcohol Consumption with Polymorphisms in Alcohol-Metabolizing Enzymes on Pancreatic Cancer Risk in Japanese," *Cancer Science* 100, no. 2 (2009): 296–302, DOI:10.1111/j.1349-7006.2008.01044.

9. Valter Longo, *The Longevity Diet* (New York: Penguin Random House, 2018).

10. Valter D. Longo and Rozalyn M. Anderson, "Nutrition, Longevity and Disease: From Molecular Mechanisms to Interventions," *Cell* 185, no. 9 (April 28, 2022): 1455–70, DOI:10.1016/j.cell.2022.04.002.

11. Fondazione Valter Longo, "Longevity Diet for Adults," n.d., viewed July 10, 2023, fondazionevalterlongo.org/longevity-diet-for-adults/?lang=en.

12. Samantha M. Solon-Biet et al., "The Ratio of Macronutrients, Not Caloric Intake, Dictates Cardiometabolic Health, Aging, and Longevity in Ad Libitum-Fed Mice," *Cell Metabolism* 19, no. 3 (March 4, 2014): 418–30, DOI:10.1016/j.cmet.2014.02.009, erratum in *Cell Metabolism* 31, no. 3 (March

3, 2020): 654, DOI:10.1016/j.cmet.2020.01.010; Morgan E. Levine et al., "Low Protein Intake Is Associated with a Major Reduction in IGF-1, Cancer, and Overall Mortality in the 65 and Younger but Not Older Population," *Cell Metabolism* 19, no 3 (March 4, 2014): 407–17, DOI:10.1016/j.cmet.2014.02.006.

13. Ying Bao et al., "Association of Nut Consumption with Total and Cause-Specific Mortality," *New England Journal of Medicine* 369, no. 21 (November 21, 2013): 2001–11, DOI:10.1056/NEJMoa1307352; Sina Naghshi et al., "Association of Total Nut, Tree Nut, Peanut, and Peanut Butter Consumption with Cancer Incidence and Mortality: A Comprehensive Systematic Review and Dose-Response Meta-Analysis of Observational Studies," *Advances in Nutrition* 12, no. 3 (2021): 793–808, DOI:10.1093/advances/nmaa152.

14. Julia Baudry et al., "Association of Frequency of Organic Food Consumption with Cancer Risk: Findings from the NutriNet-Santé Prospective Cohort Study," *JAMA Internal Medicine* 178, no. 12 (2018): 1597–606, DOI:10.1001/jamainternmed.2018.4357, erratum in *JAMA Internal Medicine* 178, no. 12 (December 1, 2018): 1732, DOI:10.1001/jamainternmed.2018 .6902.

15. Marcin Barański et al., "Higher Antioxidant and Lower Cadmium Concentrations and Lower Incidence of Pesticide Residues in Organically Grown Crops: A Systematic Literature Review and Meta-Analyses," *British Journal of Nutrition* 112, no. 5 (2014): 794–811, DOI:10.1017/S0007114514001366; Mi Ah Han, Jin Hwa Kim, and Han Soo Song, "Persistent Organic Pollutants, Pesticides, and the Risk of Thyroid Cancer: Systematic Review and Meta-Analysis," *European Journal of Cancer Prevention* 28, no. 4 (2019): 344–49, DOI:10.1097/CEJ.0000000000000481; Geneviève Van Maele-Fabry, Laurence Gamet-Payrastre, and Dominique Lison, "Household Exposure to Pesticides and Risk of Leukemia in Children and Adolescents: Updated Systematic Review and Meta-Analysis," *International Journal of Hygiene and Environmental Health* 222, no. 1 (2019): 49–67, DOI:10.1016/j.ijheh.2018 .08.004.

16. Jean A. Welsh et al., "Production-Related Contaminants (Pesticides, Antibiotics and Hormones) in Organic and Conventionally Produced Milk Samples Sold in the USA," *Public Health Nutrition* 22, no. 16 (2019): 2972–80, DOI:10.1017/S136898001900106X; Annamari Kilkkinen et al., "Antibiotic Use Predicts an Increased Risk of Cancer," *International Journal of Cancer* 123, no. 9 (2008): 2152–55, DOI:10.1002/ijc.23622; Steffanie S. Amadei and Vicente Notario, "A Significant Question in Cancer Risk and Therapy: Are Antibiotics Positive or Negative Effectors? Current Answers and Possible Alternatives," *Antibiotics* 9, no. 9 (2020): 580, DOI:10.3390/antibiotics9090580.

17. Sources about alcohol consumption:
   • Aliasghar Ahmad Kiadaliri et al., "Alcohol Drinking Cessation and the Risk of Laryngeal and Pharyngeal Cancers: A Systematic Review and Meta-Analysis," *PLOS ONE* 8, no. 3 (2013): e58158, DOI:10.1371/journal .pone.0058158.

- Christopher Griffith and Douglas Bogart, "Alcohol Consumption: Can We Safely Toast to Our Health?," *Missouri Medicine* 109, no. 6 (2012): 459–65.
- Mia Hashibe et al., "Interaction Between Tobacco and Alcohol Use and the Risk of Head and Neck Cancer: Pooled Analysis in the International Head and Neck Cancer Epidemiology Consortium," *Cancer Epidemiology, Biomarkers & Prevention* 18, no. 2 (2009): 541–50, DOI:10.1158/1055-9965.EPI-08-0347.
- Naomi E. Allen et al., "Moderate Alcohol Intake and Cancer Incidence in Women," *Journal of the National Cancer Institute* 101, no. 5 (2009): 296–305, DOI:10.1093/jnci/djn514.
- V. Bagnardi et al., "Alcohol Consumption and Site-Specific Cancer Risk: A Comprehensive Dose-Response Meta-Analysis," *British Journal of Cancer* 112, no. 3 (2015): 580–93, DOI:10.1038/bjc.2014.579.
- Noelle K. LoConte et al., "Alcohol and Cancer: A Statement of the American Society of Clinical Oncology," *Journal of Clinical Oncology* 36, no. 1 (2018): 83–93, DOI:10.1200/JCO.2017.76.1155.
- Nathalie Druesne-Pecollo et al., "Alcohol Drinking and Second Primary Cancer Risk in Patients with Upper Aerodigestive Tract Cancers: A Systematic Review and Meta-Analysis of Observational Studies," *Cancer Epidemiology, Biomarkers & Prevention* 23, no. 2 (2014): 324–31, DOI:10.1158/1055-9965.EPI-13-0779. PMID: 24307268.
- Ke Ma et al., "Alcohol Consumption and Gastric Cancer Risk: A Meta-Analysis," *Medical Science Monitor* 23 (January 2017): 238–46, DOI:10.12659/msm.899423.
- Jinhui Zhao et al., "Is Alcohol Consumption a Risk Factor for Prostate Cancer? A Systematic Review and Meta-Analysis," *BMC Cancer* 16, no. 1 (2016): 845, DOI:10.1186/s12885-016-2891-z.
- I. Tramacere et al., "Alcohol Drinking and Non-Hodgkin Lymphoma Risk: A Systematic Review and a Meta-Analysis," *Annals of Oncology* 23, no. 11 (2012): 2791–98, DOI:10.1093/annonc/mds013.
- U.S. Department of Agriculture and U.S. Department of Health and Human Services, "Dietary Guidelines for Americans, 2020–2025," December 2020, viewed July 10, 2023, DietaryGuidelines.gov.
- Kanda et al., "Impact of Alcohol Consumption."
- Chen Wu et al., "Joint Analysis of Three Genome-Wide Association Studies of Esophageal Squamous Cell Carcinoma in Chinese Populations," *Nature Genetics* 46 (2014): 1001–6, DOI:10.1038/ng.3064.

18. Christian Werner et al., "Physical Exercise Prevents Cellular Senescence in Circulating Leukocytes and in the Vessel Wall," *Circulation* 120, no. 24 (2009): 2438–47, DOI:10.1161/CIRCULATIONAHA.109.861005.
19. Brigid M. Lynch, Heather K. Neilson, and Christine M. Friedenreich, "Physical Activity and Breast Cancer Prevention," *Recent Results in Cancer Research* 186 (2011): 13–42, DOI:10.1007/978-3-642-04231-7_2.
20. G. Behrens and M. F. Leitzmann, "The Association Between Physical Activity and Renal Cancer: Systematic Review and Meta-Analysis," *British*

Journal of Cancer 108, no. 4 (2013): 798–811, DOI:10.1038/bjc.2013.37; Terry Boyle et al., "Physical Activity and Risks of Proximal and Distal Colon Cancers: A Systematic Review and Meta-Analysis," *Journal of the National Cancer Institute* 104, no. 20 (2012): 1548–61, DOI:10.1093/jnci/djs354; Jia-Yang Sun et al., "Physical Activity and Risk of Lung Cancer: A Meta-Analysis of Prospective Cohort Studies," *Asian Pacific Journal of Cancer Prevention* 13, no. 7 (2012): 3143–47, DOI:10.7314/apjcp.2012.13.7.3143; Dorien W. Voskuil et al., "Physical Activity and Endometrial Cancer Risk, a Systematic Review of Current Evidence," *Cancer Epidemiology, Biomarkers & Prevention* 16, no. 4 (2007): 639–48, DOI:10.1158/1055-9965.EPI-06-0742; YuPeng Liu et al., "Does Physical Activity Reduce the Risk of Prostate Cancer? A Systematic Review and Meta-Analysis," *European Urology* 60, no. 5 (2011): 1029–44, DOI:10.1016/j.eururo.2011.07.007.

21. Alexander Mok et al., "Physical Activity Trajectories and Mortality: Population Based Cohort Study," *British Medical Journal* 365, no. l2323 (June 29, 2019), DOI:10.1136/bmj.l2323.

22. Shahid Mahmood et al., "Domain-Specific Physical Activity and Sedentary Behaviour in Relation to Colon and Rectal Cancer Risk: A Systematic Review and Meta-Analysis," *International Journal of Epidemiology* 46, no. 6 (2017): 1797–813, DOI:10.1093/ije/dyx137. PMID: 29025130.

23. Catherine Handy Marshall et al., "Cardiorespiratory Fitness and Incident Lung and Colorectal Cancer in Men and Women: Results from the Henry Ford Exercise Testing (FIT) Cohort," *Cancer* 125, no. 15 (2019): 2594–601, DOI:10.1002/cncr.32085.

24. Carol Ewing Garber et al., "American College of Sports Medicine Position Stand. Quantity and Quality of Exercise for Developing and Maintaining Cardiorespiratory, Musculoskeletal, and Neuromotor Fitness in Apparently Healthy Adults: Guidance for Prescribing Exercise," *Medicine and Science in Sports and Exercise* 43, no. 7 (2011): 1334–59, DOI:10.1249/MSS.0b013 e318213fefb.

25. Douglas Paddon-Jones and Blake B. Rasmussen, "Dietary Protein Recommendations and the Prevention of Sarcopenia," *Current Opinion in Clinical Nutrition and Metabolic Care* 12, no. 1 (2009): 86–90, DOI:10.1097 /MCO.0b013e32831cef8b; Vinod Kumar et al., "Age-Related Differences in the Dose-Response Relationship of Muscle Protein Synthesis to Resistance Exercise in Young and Old Men," *Journal of Physiology* 587, no. 1 (2009): 211–17, DOI:10.1113/jphysiol.2008.164483.

26. Pernille Hojman et al., "Molecular Mechanisms Linking Exercise to Cancer Prevention and Treatment," *Cell Metabolism* 27, no. 1 (2018): 10–21, DOI:10.1016/j.cmet.2017.09.015.

27. Jeffrey A. Meyerhardt et al., "Randomized Phase II Trial of Exercise, Metformin, or Both on Metabolic Biomarkers in Colorectal and Breast Cancer Survivors," *JNCI Cancer Spectrum* 4, no. 1 (2019): pkz096 DOI:10.1093/jncics /pkz096.

28. Macmillan Cancer Support, "Principles and Guidance for the Prehabilitation Within the Management and Support of People with Cancer," November

30, 2020, macmillan.org.uk/healthcare-professionals/news-and-resources
/guides/principles-and-guidance-for-prehabilitation.

29. Alice Avancini et al., "Exercise Prehabilitation in Lung Cancer: Getting
Stronger to Recover Faster," *European Journal of Surgical Oncology* 47, no. 8
(March 17, 2021): 1847–55, DOI:10.1016/j.ejso.2021.03.231.

30. M. G. MacVicar, M. L. Winningham, and J. L. Nickel, "Effects of Aerobic
Interval Training on Cancer Patients' Functional Capacity," *Nursing Re-
search* 38, no. 6 (1989): 348–51; M. L. Winningham and M. G. MacVicar, "The
Effect of Aerobic Exercise on Patient Reports of Nausea," *Oncology Nursing
Forum* 15, no. 4 (1988): 4447–50; M. L. Winningham et al., "Effect of Aerobic
Exercise on Body Weight and Composition in Patients with Breast Cancer
on Adjuvant Chemotherapy," *Oncology Nursing Forum* 16, no. 5 (1989): 683–89,
PMID:2780404.

31. Kerry S. Courneya et al., "Randomized Controlled Trial of the Effects of
Aerobic Exercise on Physical Functioning and Quality of Life in Lymphoma
Patients," *Journal of Clinical Oncology* 27, no. 27 (2009): 4605–12, DOI:10.1200/
JCO.2008.20.0634; K. S. Courneya et al., "A Randomized Trial of Exercise
and Quality of Life in Colorectal Cancer Survivors," *European Journal of
Cancer Care* 12, no. 4 (2003): 347–57, DOI:10.1046/j.1365-2354.2003.00437.x;
Karen M. Mustian et al., "Exercise and Side Effects Among 749 Patients
During and After Treatment for Cancer: A University of Rochester Cancer
Center Community Clinical Oncology Program Study," *Supportive Care in
Cancer* 14, no. 7 (2006): 732–41, DOI:10.1007/s00520-005-0912-6.

32. Susan R. Harris et al., "Clinical Practice Guidelines for Breast Cancer
Rehabilitation—Syntheses of Guideline Recommendations and Qualitative Appraisals," *Cancer* 118, no. 8 suppl. (2012): 2312–24, DOI:10.1002
/cncr.27461; V. De Luca et al., "Effects of Concurrent Aerobic and Strength
Training on Breast Cancer Survivors: A Pilot Study," *Public Health* 136
(2016): 126–32, DOI:10.1016/j.puhe.2016.03.028.

33. Lynch, Neilson, and Friedenreich, "Physical Activity and Breast Cancer
Prevention."

34. P. Cormie et al., "Exercise Maintains Sexual Activity in Men Undergoing
Androgen Suppression for Prostate Cancer: A Randomized Controlled
Trial," *Prostate Cancer Prostatic Diseases* 16, no. 2 (2013): 170–75, DOI:10.1038
/pcan.2012.52.

35. Caffa et al., "Fasting-Mimicking Diet and Hormone Therapy."

36. O. Grundmann, S. L. Yoon, and J. J. Williams, "The Value of Bioelectrical
Impedance Analysis and Phase Angle in the Evaluation of Malnutrition
and Quality of Life in Cancer Patients: A Comprehensive Review," *European Journal of Clinical Nutrition* 69, no. 12 (2015): 1290–97, DOI:10.1038
/ejcn.2015.126.

37. Caffa et al., "Fasting-Mimicking Diet and Hormone Therapy."

38. Kristin L. Campbell et al., "Exercise Guidelines for Cancer Survivors: Consensus Statement from International Multidisciplinary Roundtable," *Medicine & Science in Sports & Exercise* 51, no. 11 (November 2019): 2375–90,
DOI:10.1249/MSS.0000000000002116.

4. FASTING, NUTRITION, AND BREAST CANCER

1. National Cancer Institute, "Advances in Breast Cancer Research," n.d., viewed July 10, 2023, cancer.gov/types/breast/research.
2. Darlan C. Minussi et al., "Breast Tumours Maintain a Reservoir of Subclonal Diversity During Expansion," *Nature* 592 (2021): 302–8, DOI:10.1038/s41586-021-03357-x.
3. Salvatore Cortellino et al., "Fasting Renders Immunotherapy Effective Against Low-Immunogenic Breast Cancer While Reducing Side Effects," *Cell Reports* 40, no. 8 (August 23, 2022): 111256, DOI:10.1016/j.celrep.2022.111256.
4. Stefanie de Groot et al., "The Effects of Short-Term Fasting on Tolerance to (Neo) Adjuvant Chemotherapy in HER2-Negative Breast Cancer Patients: A Randomized Pilot Study," *BMC Cancer* 15 (2015): 625, DOI:10.1186/s12885-015-1663-5.
5. Stephan P. Bauersfeld et al., "The Effects of Short-Term Fasting on Quality of Life and Tolerance to Chemotherapy in Patients with Breast and Ovarian Cancer: A Randomized Cross-Over Pilot Study," *BMC Cancer* 18, no. 1 (2018): 476, DOI:10.1186/s12885-018-4353-2.
6. Stefano Di Biase et al., "Fasting Regulates EGR1 and Protects from Glucose- and Dexamethasone-Dependent Sensitization to Chemotherapy," *PLOS Biology* 15, no. 3 (2017): e2001951, DOI:10.1371/journal.pbio.2001951, correction in *PLOS Biology* 15, no. 5 (May 1, 2017): e1002603.
7. de Groot et al., "Effects of Short-Term Fasting."
8. Irene Caffa et al., "Fasting-Mimicking Diet and Hormone Therapy Induce Breast Cancer Regression," *Nature* 583, no. 7817 (July 2020): 620–24, DOI:10.1038/s41586-020-2502-7, author correction in *Nature* 588, no. 7839 (December 2020): E33.
9. Francesca Ligorio et al., "Adding Fasting-Mimicking Diet to First-Line Carboplatin-Based Chemotherapy Is Associated with Better Overall Survival in Advanced Triple-Negative Breast Cancer Patients: A Subanalysis of the NCT03340935 Trial," *International Journal of Cancer* 154, no. 1 (2024): 114–23, DOI:10.1002/ijc.34701.
10. Stefanie Zorn et al., "Impact of Modified Short-Term Fasting and Its Combination with a Fasting Supportive Diet During Chemotherapy on the Incidence and Severity of Chemotherapy-Induced Toxicities in Cancer Patients—A Controlled Cross-Over Pilot Study," *BMC Cancer* 20, no. 1 (2020): 578, DOI:10.1186/s12885-020-07041-7.
11. Philippine Fassier et al., "Fasting and Weight-Loss Restrictive Diet Practices Among 2,700 Cancer Survivors: Results from the NutriNet-Santé Cohort," *International Journal of Cancer* 143, no. 11 (2018): 2687–97, DOI:10.1002/ijc.31646.
12. Sébastien Mas, Alice Le Bonniec, and Florence Cousson-Gélie, "Why Do Women Fast During Breast Cancer Chemotherapy? A Qualitative Study of the Patient Experience," *British Journal of Health Psychology* 24, no. 2 (2019): 381–95, DOI:10.1111/bjhp.12358.
13. Francesca Valdemarin et al., "Safety and Feasibility of Fasting-Mimicking Diet and Effects on Nutritional Status and Circulating Metabolic and In-

flammatory Factors in Cancer Patients Undergoing Active Treatment," *Cancers (Basel)* 13, no. 16 (August 9, 2021): 4013, DOI:10.3390/cancers13164013; Claudio Vernieri et al., "Fasting-Mimicking Diet Is Safe and Reshapes Metabolism and Antitumor Immunity in Patients with Cancer," *Cancer Discovery* 12, no. 1 (January 2022): 90–107, DOI:10.1158/2159-8290.CD-21-0030.

14. Francesca Ligorio et al., "Exceptional Tumour Responses to Fasting-Mimicking Diet Combined with Standard Anticancer Therapies: A Sub-Analysis of the NCT03340935 Trial," *European Journal of Cancer* 172 (September 2022): 300–310, DOI:10.1016/j.ejca.2022.05.046.

15. Giulia Salvadori et al., "Fasting-Mimicking Diet Blocks Triple-Negative Breast Cancer and Cancer Stem Cell Escape," *Cell Metabolism* 33, no. 11 (2021): 2247–59, DOI:10.1016/j.cmet.2021.10.008.

16. Caffa et al., "Fasting-Mimicking Diet and Hormone Therapy."

17. Ligorio et al., "Exceptional Tumour Responses."

18. Paolo Contiero et al., "Fasting Blood Glucose and Long-Term Prognosis of Non-Metastatic Breast Cancer: A Cohort Study," *Breast Cancer Research and Treatment* 138, no. 3 (2013): 951–59, DOI:10.1007/s10549-013-2519-9.

19. Catherine R. Marinac et al., "Prolonged Nightly Fasting and Breast Cancer Prognosis," *JAMA Oncology* 2, no. 8 (2016): 1049–55, DOI:10.1001/jamaoncol.2016.0164.

20. Anne T. Berg et al., "How Long Does It Take for Epilepsy to Become Intractable? A Prospective Investigation," *Annals of Neurology* 60, no. 1 (2006): 73–79, DOI:10.1002/ana.20852.

21. Alessio Nencioni et al., "Fasting and Cancer: Molecular Mechanisms and Clinical Application," *Nature Reviews Cancer* 18, no. 11 (2018): 707–19, DOI:10.1038/s41568-018-0061-0.

22. Adeleh Khodabakhshi et al., "Feasibility, Safety, and Beneficial Effects of MCT-Based Ketogenic Diet for Breast Cancer Treatment: A Randomized Controlled Trial Study," *Clinical Nutrition* 40, no. 3 (2021): 751–58, DOI:10.1016/j.clnu.2020.06.028.

23. Adeleh Khodabakhshi et al., "Effects of Ketogenic Metabolic Therapy on Patients with Breast Cancer: A Randomized Controlled Clinical Trial," *Clinical Nutrition 40, no. 3 (2021): 751–58.*

24. Nencioni et al., "Fasting and Cancer."

5. FASTING, NUTRITION, AND GYNECOLOGICAL CANCERS

1. National Center for Chronic Disease Prevention and Health Promotion (U.S.), Division of Cancer Prevention and Control, "Gynecologic Cancer Incidence, United States—2012–2016," United States cancer statistics data brief; no. 11, September 2019, https://stacks.cdc.gov/view/cdc/81916.

2. World Cancer Research Fund International, "Ovarian Cancer Statistics," n.d., viewed July 10, 2023, wcrf.org/dietandcancer/cancer-trends/ovarian-cancer-statistics.

3. World Cancer Research Fund International, "Cervical Cancer Statistics," n.d., viewed July 10, 2023, wcrf.org/dietandcancer/cancer-trends/cervical-cancer-statistics.

4. World Cancer Research Fund International, "Endometrial Cancer Statistics," n.d., viewed July 10, 2023, wcrf.org/cancer-trends/endometrial-cancer-statistics/.

5. Kathleen Moore et al., "Maintenance Olaparib in Patients with Newly Diagnosed Advanced Ovarian Cancer," *New England Journal of Medicine* 379 (2018); 2495–505, DOI:10.1056/NEJMoa1810858; Antonio González-Martín et al., "Niraparib in Patients with Newly Diagnosed Advanced Ovarian Cancer," *New England Journal of Medicine* 381 (2019): 2391–402, DOI:10.1056/NEJMoa1910962; Isabelle Ray-Coquard et al., "Olaparib Plus Bevacizumab as First-Line Maintenance in Ovarian Cancer," *New England Journal of Medicine* 381 (2019): 2416–28, DOI:10.1056/NEJMoa1911361.

6. Nicole Concin et al., "ESGO/ESTRO/ESP Guidelines for the Management of Patients with Endometrial Carcinoma," *Radiotherapy & Oncology* 154 (2021): 327–53, DOI:10.1016/j.radonc.2020.11.018.

7. Changhan Lee et al., "Fasting Cycles Retard Growth of Tumors and Sensitize a Range of Cancer Cell Types to Chemotherapy," *Science Translational Medicine* 4, no. 124 (2012): 124ra27, DOI:10.1126/scitranslmed.3003293.

8. Irene Caffa et al., "Fasting-Mimicking Diet and Hormone Therapy Induce Breast Cancer Regression," *Nature* 583, no. 7817 (2020): 620–24, DOI:10.1038/s41586-020-2502-7, author correction in *Nature* 588, no. 7839 (December 2020): E33.

9. Lizzia Raffaghello et al., "Starvation-Dependent Differential Stress Resistance Protects Normal but Not Cancer Cells Against High-Dose Chemotherapy," *Proceedings of the National Academy of Sciences of the United States of America* 105, no. 24 (June 17, 2008): 8215–20, DOI:10.1073/pnas.0708100105.

10. Fernando M. Safdie et al., "Fasting and Cancer Treatment in Humans: A Case Series Report," *Aging* 1, no. 12 (2009): 988–1007, DOI:10.18632/aging.100114.

11. Tanya B. Dorff et al., "Safety and Feasibility of Fasting in Combination with Platinum-Based Chemotherapy," *BMC Cancer* 16 (2016): 360, DOI:10.1186/s12885-016-2370-6.

12. Courtney J. Riedinger et al., "Water Only Fasting and Its Effect on Chemotherapy Administration in Gynecologic Malignancies," *Gynecologic Oncology* 159, no. 3 (December 2020): 799–803, DOI:10.1016/j.ygyno.2020.09.008.

13. Stefanie Zorn et al., "Impact of Modified Short-Term Fasting and Its Combination with a Fasting Supportive Diet During Chemotherapy on the Incidence and Severity of Chemotherapy-Induced Toxicities in Cancer Patients—A Controlled Cross-Over Pilot Study," *BMC Cancer* 20, no. 1 (June 22, 2020): 578, DOI:10.1186/s12885-020-07041-7.

14. Zorn et al., "Impact of Modified Short-Term Fasting."

15. Anke Smits et al. "The Effect of Lifestyle Interventions on the Quality of Life of Gynaecological Cancer Survivors: A Systematic Review and Meta-Analysis," *Gynecologic Oncology* 139, no. 3 (2015): 546–52, DOI:10.1016/j.ygyno.2015.10.002

16. Caroline W. Cohen et al., "A Ketogenic Diet Reduces Central Obesity and Serum Insulin in Women with Ovarian or Endometrial Cancer," *Journal of Nutrition* 148, no. 8 (2018): 1253–60, DOI:10.1093/jn/nxy119.

17. Caroline W. Cohen et al., "A Ketogenic Diet Is Acceptable in Women with Ovarian and Endometrial Cancer and Has No Adverse Effects on Blood Lipids: A Randomized, Controlled Trial," *Nutrition and Cancer* 72, no. 4 (2020): 584–94, DOI:10.1080/01635581.2019.1645864.

6. FASTING, NUTRITION, AND PROSTATE CANCER

1. World Cancer Research Fund International, "Prostate Cancer Statistics," n.d., viewed July 12, 2023, wcrf.org/dietandcancer/cancer-trends/prostate -cancer-statistics.

2. Lars Egevad et al., "International Society of Urological Pathology (ISUP) Grading of Prostate Cancer—An ISUP Consensus on Contemporary Grading," *APMIS* 124, no. 6 (June 2016): 433–35, DOI:10.1111/apm.12533.

3. National Cancer Institute, "Prostate-Specific Antigen (PSA) Test," last updated March 11, 2022, cancer.gov/types/prostate/psa-fact-sheet.

4. David L. McCormick et al., "Null Effect of Dietary Restriction on Prostate Carcinogenesis in the Wistar-Unilever Rat," *Nutrition and Cancer* 57, no. 2 (2007): 194–200, DOI:10.1080/01635580701277494.

5. Melissa J. L. Bonorden et al., "Intermittent Calorie Restriction Delays Prostate Tumor Detection and Increases Survival Time in TRAMP Mice," *Nutrition and Cancer* 61, no. 2 (2009): 265–75, DOI:10.1080/016355 80802419798.

6. W. Cooper Buschemeyer 3rd et al., "Effect of Intermittent Fasting with or Without Caloric Restriction on Prostate Cancer Growth and Survival in SCID Mice," *Prostate* 70, no. 10 (July 1, 2010): 1037–43, DOI:10.1002/pros .21136.

7. D. S. Coffey, "Similarities of Prostate and Breast Cancer: Evolution, Diet, and Estrogens," *Urology*, 57, no. 4 suppl. 1 (2001): 31–38, DOI:10.1016/s0090 -4295(00)00938-9.

8. Susanne M. Henning et al., "Phase II Prospective Randomized Trial of Weight Loss Prior to Radical Prostatectomy," *Prostate Cancer and Prostatic Disease* 21, no. 2 (2018): 212–20, DOI:10.1038/s41391-017-0001-1.

9. Erez Eitan et al., "In a Randomized Trial in Prostate Cancer Patients, Dietary Protein Restriction Modifies Markers of Leptin and Insulin Signaling in Plasma Extracellular Vesicles," *Aging Cell* 16, no. 6 (December 2017): 1430–33, DOI:10.1111/acel.12657.

10. Stephen J. Freedland et al., "A Randomized Controlled Trial of a 6-Month Low-Carbohydrate Intervention on Disease Progression in Men with Recurrent Prostate Cancer: Carbohydrate and Prostate Study 2 (CAPS2)," *Clinical Cancer Research* 26, no. 12 (June 15, 2020): 3035–43, DOI:10.1158/1078 -0432.CCR-19-3873.

11. Sajjad Moradi et al., "Associations Between Dietary Inflammatory Index and Incidence of Breast and Prostate Cancer: A Systematic Review and

Meta-Analysis," *Nutrition* 55–56 (November 2018): 168–78, DOI:10.1016/j .nut.2018.04.018.

7. FASTING, NUTRITION, AND COLORECTAL CANCER

1. World Cancer Research Fund International, "Colorectal Cancer Statistics," n.d., viewed July 12, 2023, wcrf.org/dietandcancer/cancer-trends/colorectal -cancer-statistics.
2. Changhan Lee et al., "Fasting Cycles Retard Growth of Tumors and Sensitize a Range of Cancer Cell Types to Chemotherapy," *Science Translational Medicine* 4, no. 124 (2012): 124ra27, DOI:10.1126/scitranslmed.3003293.
3. Irene Caffa et al., "Fasting Potentiates the Anticancer Activity of Tyrosine Kinase Inhibitors by Strengthening MAPK Signaling Inhibition," *Oncotarget* 6, no. 14 (May 20, 2015): 11820–32, DOI:10.18632/oncotarget.3689.
4. Jihye Yun et al., "Vitamin C Selectively Kills KRAS and BRAF Mutant Colorectal Cancer Cells by Targeting GAPDH," *Science* 350, no. 6266 (December 11, 2015): 1391–96, DOI:10.1126/science.aaa5004.
5. National Cancer Institute, "Researchers Discover Potential Way to Hit Elusive Target in Pancreatic Cancer," April 4, 2019, cancer.gov/news-events /cancer-currents-blog/2019/pancreatic-cancer-targeting-kras-indirectly.
6. Maira Di Tano et al., "Synergistic Effect of Fasting-Mimicking Diet and Vitamin C Against KRAS Mutated Cancers," *Nature Communications* 11, no. 1 (May 11, 2020): 2332, DOI:10.1038/s41467-020-16243-3.
7. M. L. Weng et al. "Fasting Inhibits Aerobic Glycolysis and Proliferation in Colorectal Cancer via the Fdft1-mediated AKT/mTOR/HIF1α Pathway Suppression," *Nature Communications* 11, no. 1 (April 20, 2020): 1869, DOI: 10.1038/s41467-020-15795-8.
8. Stefano Di Biase et al., "Fasting Regulates EGR1 and Protects from Glucose- and Dexamethasone-Dependent Sensitization to Chemotherapy," *PLOS Biology* 15, no. 3 (March 30, 2017): e2001951, DOI:10.1371/journal.pbio.2001951, correction in *PLOS Biology* 15, no. 5 (May 1, 2017): e1002603.
9. "Effects of Fasting Strategies on Postoperative Recovery and Long-Term Prognosis in Patients with Colorectal Cancer," NCT04345978, clinicaltrials. gov/study/NCT04345978.
10. "Short-Term Fasting as an Enhancer of Chemotherapy: Pilot Clinical Study on Colorectal Carcinoma Patients (CHEMOFAST)," NCT04247464, clinicaltrials.gov/study/NCT04247464.
11. Marta Borges-Canha et al., "Role of Colonic Microbiota in Colorectal Carcinogenesis: A Systematic Review," *Revista española de enfermedades digestivas* 107, no. 11 (November 2015): 659–71, DOI:10.17235/reed.2015.3830 /2015.
12. Lidia Sánchez-Alcoholado et al., "The Role of the Gut Microbiome in Colorectal Cancer Development and Therapy Response," *Cancers* 12, no. 6 (May 29, 2020):1406, DOI:10.3390/cancers12061406.
13. Stephen J. D. O'Keefe et al., "Fat, Fibre and Cancer Risk in African Americans and Rural Africans," *Nature Communications* 6 (2015): 6342, DOI:10 .1038/ncomms7342.

14. Erin L. Van Blarigan et al., "Association of Survival with Adherence to the American Cancer Society Nutrition and Physical Activity Guidelines for Cancer Survivors After Colon Cancer Diagnosis: The CALGB 89803/Alliance Trial," *JAMA Oncology* 4, no. 6 (2018): 783–90, DOI:10.1001/jamaoncol .2018.0126.

15. Shivtaj Mann, Manreet Sidhu, and Krisstina Gowin, "Understanding the Mechanisms of Diet and Outcomes in Colon, Prostate, and Breast Cancer; Malignant Gliomas; and Cancer Patients on Immunotherapy," *Nutrients* 12, no. 8 (July 26, 2020): 2226, DOI:10.3390/nu12082226.

16. Muhammad-Afiq Osman et al., "16S rRNA Gene Sequencing for Deciphering the Colorectal Cancer Gut Microbiome: Current Protocols and Workflows," *Frontiers in Microbiology* 9 (April 2018): 767, DOI:10.3389 /fmicb.2018.00767.

17. Francesca Ligorio et al., "Exceptional Tumour Responses to Fasting-Mimicking Diet Combined with Standard Anticancer Therapies: A Sub-Analysis of the NCT03340935 Trial," *European Journal of Cancer* 172 (September 2022): 300–310, DOI:10.1016/j.ejca.2022.05.046.

8. FASTING, NUTRITION, AND LUNG CANCER

1. American Cancer Society, "Key Statistics for Lung Cancer," last revised January 12, 2023, cancer.org/cancer/lung-cancer/about/key-statistics.html.

2. Centers for Disease Control and Prevention, "Lung Cancer Risk Factors," November 7, 2023, https://www.cdc.gov/lung-cancer/risk-factors/?CDC _AAref_Val=https://www.cdc.gov/cancer/lung/basic_info/risk_factors .htm.

3. Hilary A. Tindle et al., "Lifetime Smoking History and Risk of Lung Cancer: Results From the Framingham Heart Study," *Journal of the National Cancer Institute* 110, no. 11 (2018): 1201–7, DOI:10.1093/jnci/djy041.

4. American Cancer Society, "Lung Cancer Risk Factors," n.d., last revised November 20, 2023, cancer.org/cancer/lung-cancer/causes-risks-prevention /risk-factors.html.

5. Robert Pirker, "Adjuvant Chemotherapy in Patients with Completely Resected Non-Small Cell Lung Cancer," *Translational Lung Cancer Research* 3, no. 5 (2014): 305–10, DOI:10.3978/j.issn.2218-6751.2014.09.13.

6. Yandong Shi et al., "Starvation-Induced Activation of ATM/Chk2/P53 Signaling Sensitizes Cancer Cells to Cisplatin," *BMC Cancer* 12 (2012): 571, DOI:10.1186/1471-2407-12-571.

7. Irene Caffa et al., "Fasting Potentiates the Anticancer Activity of Tyrosine Kinase Inhibitors by Strengthening MAPK Signaling Inhibition," *Oncotarget* 6, no. 14 (2015): 11820–32, DOI:10.18632/oncotarget.3689.

8. Giulia Salvadori et al., "Fasting-Mimicking Diet Blocks Triple-Negative Breast Cancer and Cancer Stem Cell Escape," *Cell Metabolism* 33, no. 11 (2021): 2247–59, DOI:10.1016/j.cmet.2021.10.008.

9. Maira Di Tano et al., "Synergistic Effect of Fasting-Mimicking Diet and Vitamin C Against KRAS Mutated Cancers," *Nature Communications* 11, no. 1 (2020): 2332, DOI:10.1038/s41467-020-16243-3.

10. Stefano Di Biase et al., "Fasting-Mimicking Diet Reduces HO-1 to Promote T Cell–Mediated Tumor Cytotoxicity," *Cancer Cell* 30, no. 1 (2016): 136–46, DOI:10.1016/j.ccell.2016.06.005.
11. Claudio Vernieri et al., "Fasting-Mimicking Diet Is Safe and Reshapes Metabolism and Antitumor Immunity in Patients with Cancer," *Cancer Discovery* 12, no. 1 (January 2022): 90–107, DOI:10.1158/2159-8290.CD-21-0030.
12. Daniel Ajona et al., "Short-Term Starvation Reduces IGF-1 Levels to Sensitize Lung Tumors to PD-1 Immune Checkpoint Blockade," *Nature Cancer* 1 (2020): 75–85, DOI:10.1038/s43018-019-0007-9.
13. Fernando M. Safdie et al., "Fasting and Cancer Treatment in Humans: A Case Series Report," *Aging* 1, no. 12 (2009): 988–1007, DOI:10.18632/aging.100114.
14. Francesca Ligorio et al., "Exceptional Tumour Responses to Fasting-Mimicking Diet Combined with Standard Anticancer Therapies: A Sub-Analysis of the NCT03340935 Trial," *European Journal of Cancer* 172 (September 2022): 300–10, DOI:10.1016/j.ejca.2022.05.046.
15. Francesca Valdemarin et al., "Safety and Feasibility of Fasting-Mimicking Diet and Effects on Nutritional Status and Circulating Metabolic and Inflammatory Factors in Cancer Patients Undergoing Active Treatment," *Cancers* 13, no. 6 (August 9, 2021): 4013, DOI:10.3390/cancers13164013.
16. Ligorio et al., "Exceptional Tumour Responses."
17. Juhua Luo, Yea-Jyh Chen, and Li-Jung Chang, "Fasting Blood Glucose Level and Prognosis in Non-Small-Cell Lung Cancer (NSCLC) Patients," *Lung Cancer* 76, no. 2 (2012): 242–47, DOI:10.1016/j.lungcan.2011.10.019.
18. Jin-Rong Yang et al., "Fasting Blood Glucose Levels and Prognosis in Patients with Non-Small-Cell Lung Cancer: A Prospective Cohort Study in China," *OncoTargets and Therapy* 12 (July 23, 2019): 5947–53, DOI:10.2147/OTT.S210103.
19. "Randomized Controlled Pilot Study to Evaluate Fasting-Mimicking Diet in Patients Receiving Chemo-Immunotherapy for Treatment of Metastatic Non-Small Cell Lung Cancer," 1807475941 (IUSCC-0662), https://research-studies.allinforhealth.info/us/en/listing/1427/randomized-controlled-pilot-study/.
20. Amir Zahra et al., "Consuming a Ketogenic Diet While Receiving Radiation and Chemotherapy for Locally Advanced Lung Cancer and Pancreatic Cancer: The University of Iowa Experience of Two Phase 1 Clinical Trials," *Radiation Research* 187, no. 6 (2017): 743–54, DOI:10.1667/RR14668.1.
21. Karla Sánchez-Lara et al., "Effects of an Oral Nutritional Supplement Containing Eicosapentaenoic Acid on Nutritional and Clinical Outcomes in Patients with Advanced Non–Small Cell Lung Cancer: Randomised Trial," *Clinical Nutrition* 33, no. 6 (2014): 1017–23, DOI:10.1016/j.clnu.2014.03.006.
22. Tadashi Akiba et al., "Vitamin D Supplementation and Survival of Patients with Non–Small Cell Lung Cancer: A Randomized, Double-Blind, Placebo-Controlled Trial," *Clinical Cancer Research* 24, no. 17 (September 1, 2018): 4089–97, DOI:10.1158/1078-0432.CCR-18-0483.

9. FASTING, NUTRITION, AND BLOOD CANCERS

1. National Cancer Institute, "Hematologic Cancer," n.d., viewed on July 14, 2023, cancer.gov/publications/dictionaries/cancer-terms/def/hematologic -cancer.

2. Mayo Clinic, "Leukemia," n.d., viewed on July 14, 2023, mayoclinic.org /diseases-conditions/leukemia/diagnosis-treatment/drc-20374378; City of Hope, "Blood Cancer," n.d., last updated June 21, 2023, cancercenter.com /blood-cancers.

3. Sebastian Brandhorst et al., "A Periodic Diet That Mimics Fasting Promotes Multi-System Regeneration, Enhanced Cognitive Performance, and Healthspan," *Cell Metabolism* 22, no. 1 (2015): 86–99, DOI:10.1016/j.cmet .2015.05.012.

4. Zhigang Lu et al., "Fasting Selectively Blocks Development of Acute Lymphoblastic Leukemia via Leptin-Receptor Upregulation," *Nature Medicine* 23, no. 1 (January 2017): 79–90, DOI:10.1038/nm.4252.

5. Lu et al., "Fasting Selectively Blocks."

6. Toshia R. Myers, Mary Zittel, and Alan C. Goldhamer, "Follow-Up of Water-Only Fasting and an Exclusively Plant Food Diet in the Management of Stage IIIa, Low-Grade Follicular Lymphoma," *BMJ Case Reports* 2018 (August 9, 2018): bcr2018225520, DOI:10.1136/bcr-2018-225520.

7. Myers, Zittel, and Goldhamer, "Follow-Up of Water-Only Fasting."

8. Amelia Maria Gaman et al., "The Role of Oxidative Stress and the Effects of Antioxidants on the Incidence of Infectious Complications of Chronic Lymphocytic Leukemia," *Oxidative Medicine and Cellular Longevity* 2014 (2014): 158135, DOI:10.1155/2014/158135.

9. Xuesong Han et al., "Vegetable and Fruit Intake and Non-Hodgkin Lymphoma Survival in Connecticut Women," *Leukemia & Lymphoma* 51, no. 6 (June 2010): 1047–54, DOI:10.3109/10428191003690364.

10. FASTING, NUTRITION, AND BRAIN CANCER

1. Ahmad Faleh Tamimi and Malik Juweid, "Epidemiology and Outcome of Glioblastoma," in *Glioblastoma*, Steven De Vleeschouwer, ed. (Brisbane, Australia: Codon, 2017), available at ncbi.nlm.nih.gov/books/NBK470003/.

2. Fernando Safdie et al., "Fasting Enhances the Response of Glioma to Chemo- and Radiotherapy," *PLOS ONE* 7, no. 9 (2012): e44603, DOI:10.1371 /journal.pone.0044603.

3. Martin Voss et al., "ERGO2: A Prospective, Randomized Trial of Caloric Restricted Ketogenic Diet and Fasting in Addition to Reirradiation for Malignant Glioma," *International Journal of Radiation Oncology, Biology, Physics* 108, no. 4 (2020): 987–95, DOI:10.1016/j.ijrobp.2020.06.021.

4. Giulio Zuccoli et al., "Metabolic Management of Glioblastoma Multiforme Using Standard Therapy Together with a Restricted Ketogenic Diet: Case Report," *Nutrition & Metabolism* 7 (2010): 33, DOI:10.1186/1743 -7075-7-33.

5. Ahmed M. A. Elsakka et al., "Management of Glioblastoma Multiforme in a Patient Treated with Ketogenic Metabolic Therapy and Modified Standard of Care: A 24-Month Follow-up," *Frontiers in Nutrition* 5, no. 20 (2018), DOI:10.3389/fnut.2018.00020.

6. Johannes Rieger et al., "ERGO: A Pilot Study of Ketogenic Diet in Recurrent Glioblastoma," *International Journal of Oncology* 44, no. 6 (2014): 1843–52, DOI:10.3892/ijo.2014.2382.

7. Kenneth Schwartz et al., "Treatment of Glioma Patients with Ketogenic Diets: Report of Two Cases Treated with an IRB-Approved Energy-Restricted Ketogenic Diet Protocol and Review of the Literature," *Cancer & Metabolism* 3, no. 3 (2015), DOI:10.1186/s40170-015-0129-1.

8. Kirsty J. Martin-McGill et al., "Ketogenic Diets as an Adjuvant Therapy in Glioblastoma (the KEATING Trial): Study Protocol for a Randomised Pilot Study," *Pilot and Feasibility Studies* 3 (2017): 67, DOI:10.1186/s40814-017-0209-9.

9. Kirsty J. Martin-McGill et al., "Ketogenic Diets as an Adjuvant Therapy for Glioblastoma (KEATING): A Randomized, Mixed Methods, Feasibility Study," *Journal of Neuro-Oncology* 147, no. 1 (2020): 213–27, DOI:10.1007/s11060-020-03417-8.

10. Elles J.T.M. van der Louw et al., "Ketogenic Diet Treatment as Adjuvant to Standard Treatment of Glioblastoma Multiforme: A Feasibility and Safety Study," *Therapeutic Advances in Medical Oncology* 11 (2019): 1758835919853958, DOI:10.1177/1758835919853958.

11. Pavel Klein et al., "Treatment of Glioblastoma Multiforme with 'Classic' 4:1 Ketogenic Diet Total Meal Replacement," *Cancer & Metabolism* 8, no. 1 (2020): 24, DOI:10.1186/s40170-020-00230-9.

11. FASTING, NUTRITION, AND SKIN CANCER

1. World Cancer Research Fund International, "Skin Cancer Statistics," n.d., viewed July 14, 2023, wcrf.org/ dietandcancer/skin-cancer-statistics; International Agency for Research on Cancer (World Health Organization), "Skin Cancer," n.d., viewed July 14, 2023, iarc.who.int/cancer-type/skin-cancer/.

2. National Collaborating Centre for Cancer (UK), "Staging of Melanoma," in *Melanoma: Assessment and Management* (NICE Guideline, No. 14) (London: National Institute for Health and Care Excellence (UK), 2015), available at ncbi.nlm.nih.gov/books/NBK338424/.

3. Morgan E. Levine et al., "Low Protein Intake Is Associated with a Major Reduction in IGF-1, Cancer, and Overall Mortality in the 65 and Younger but Not Older Population," *Cell Metabolism* 19, no. 3 (March 4, 2014): 407–17, DOI:10.1016/j.cmet.2014.02.006.

4. Hong Seok Shim et al., "Starvation Promotes REV1 SUMOylation and p53-Dependent Sensitization of Melanoma and Breast Cancer Cells," *Cancer Research* 75, no. 6 (2015): 1056–67, DOI:10.1158/0008-5472.CAN-14-2249.

5. Changhan Lee et al., "Fasting Cycles Retard Growth of Tumors and Sensitize a Range of Cancer Cell Types to Chemotherapy," *Science Translational Medicine* 4, no. 124 (2012): 124ra27, DOI:10.1126/scitranslmed.3003293.
6. Lee et al., "Fasting Cycles Retard Growth."
7. Sebastian Brandhorst et al., "A Periodic Diet That Mimics Fasting Promotes Multi-System Regeneration, Enhanced Cognitive Performance, and Healthspan," *Cell Metabolism* 22, no. 1 (2015): 86–99, DOI:10.1016/j.cmet.2015.05.012.
8. Fernanda Antunes et al., "Effective Synergy of Sorafenib and Nutrient Shortage in Inducing Melanoma Cell Death Through Energy Stress," *Cells* 9, no. 3 (March 6, 2020): 640, DOI:10.3390/cells9030640.
9. Junna Oba et al., "Elevated Serum Leptin Levels Are Associated with an Increased Risk of Sentinel Lymph Node Metastasis in Cutaneous Melanoma," *Medicine* 95, no. 11 (2016): e3073, DOI:10.1097/MD.0000000000003073.

12. FASTING, NUTRITION, AND KIDNEY CANCER

1. World Cancer Research Fund International, "Kidney Cancer Statistics," n.d., viewed July 14, 2023, wcrf.org/dietandcancer/cancer-trends/kidney-cancer-statistics.
2. Wong-Ho Chow, Linda M. Dong, and Susan S. Devesa, "Epidemiology and Risk Factors for Kidney Cancer," *Nature Reviews Urology* 7, no. 5 (May 2010): 245–57, DOI:10.1038/nrurol.2010.46.
3. Donald W. Kufe et al., eds., *Holland-Frei Cancer Medicine*, 6th ed. (Hamilton, ON: BC Decker; 2003).
4. Nivedita Chowdhury and Charles G. Drake, "Kidney Cancer: An Overview of Current Therapeutic Approaches," *Urology Clinics of North America* 47, no. 4 (November 2020): 419–31, DOI:10.1016/j.ucl.2020.07.009.
5. Laura M. Lashinger et al., "Starving Cancer from the Outside and Inside: Separate and Combined Effects of Calorie Restriction and Autophagy Inhibition on Ras-Driven Tumors," *Cancer & Metabolism* 4 (September 2016): 18, DOI:10.1186/s40170-016-0158-4.
6. "Ketogenic Diet for Patients Receiving First Line Treatment for Metastatic Renal Cell Carcinoma (CETOREIN)," NCT04316520, clinicaltrials.gov/ct2/show/NCT04316520.

APPENDIX 1: MALNUTRITION SCREENING AND ASSESSMENT IN PATIENTS WITH CANCER (FOR HEALTH-CARE PROFESSIONALS)

1. Lisa Martin et al., "Assessment of Computed Tomography (CT)–Defined Muscle and Adipose Tissue Features in Relation to Short-Term Outcomes After Elective Surgery for Colorectal Cancer: A Multicenter Approach," *Annals of Surgical Oncology* 25, no. 9 (September 2018): 2669–80, DOI:10.1245/s10434-018-6652-x.
2. Miroslav Kovarik, Miroslav Hronek, and Zdenek Zadak, "Clinically Relevant Determinants of Body Composition, Function and Nutritional Status as Mortality Predictors in Lung Cancer Patients," *Lung Cancer* 84, no. 1

(April 2014): 1–6, DOI:10.1016/j.lungcan.2014.01.020; Chris Burtin et al., "Handgrip Weakness, Low Fat-Free Mass, and Overall Survival in Non–Small Cell Lung Cancer Treated with Curative-Intent Radiotherapy," *Journal of Cachexia, Sarcopenia and Muscle* 11, no. 2 (April 2020): 424–31, DOI:10.1002/jcsm.12526.

3. Lisa Martin et al., "Diagnostic Criteria for the Classification of Cancer-Associated Weight Loss," *Journal of Clinical Oncology* 33, no. 1 (January 1, 2015): 90–99, DOI:10.1200/JCO.2014.56.1894.

APPENDIX 2: FASTING AND FASTING-MIMICKING DIET CLINICAL STUDIES DURING CANCER TREATMENT

1. Min Wei et al., "Fasting-Mimicking Diet and Markers/Risk Factors for Aging, Diabetes, Cancer, and Cardiovascular Disease," *Science Translational Medicine* 9, no. 377 (February 15, 2017): eaai8700, DOI:10.1126/scitranslmed.aai8700.

2. Fernando M. Safdie et al., "Fasting and Cancer Treatment in Humans: A Case Series Report," *Aging* 1, no. 12 (December 31, 2009): 988–1007, DOI:10.18632/aging.100114.

3. Stefanie de Groot et al., "The Effects of Short-Term Fasting on Tolerance to (Neo) Adjuvant Chemotherapy in HER2-Negative Breast Cancer Patients: A Randomized Pilot Study," *BMC Cancer* 15 (October 5, 2015): 652, DOI:10.1186/s12885-015-1663-5.

4. Tanya B. Dorff et al., "Safety and Feasibility of Fasting in Combination with Platinum-Based Chemotherapy," *BMC Cancer* 16 (June 10, 2016): 360, DOI:10.1186/s12885-016-2370-6.

5. Stephan P. Bauersfeld et al., "The Effects of Short-Term Fasting on Quality of Life and Tolerance to Chemotherapy in Patients with Breast and Ovarian Cancer: A Randomized Cross-Over Pilot Study," *BMC Cancer* 18, no. 1 (April 27, 2018): 476, DOI:10.1186/s12885-018-4353-2.

6. Toshia R. Myers, Mary Zittel, and Alan C. Goldhamer, "Follow-Up of Water-Only Fasting and an Exclusively Plant Food Diet in the Management of Stage IIIa, Low-Grade Follicular Lymphoma," *BMJ Case Reports* 2018 (August 9, 2018): bcr2018225520, DOI:10.1136/bcr-2018-225520.

7. Philippine Fassier et al., "Fasting and Weight-Loss Restrictive Diet Practices Among 2,700 Cancer Survivors: Results from the NutriNet-Santé Cohort," *International Journal of Cancer* 143, no. 11 (December 1, 2018): 2687–97, DOI:10.1002/ijc.31646.

8. Sébastien Mas, Alice Le Bonniec, and Florence Cousson-Gélie, "Why Do Women Fast During Breast Cancer Chemotherapy? A Qualitative Study of the Patient Experience," *British Journal of Health Psychology* 24, no. 2 (May 2019): 381–95, DOI:10.1111/bjhp.12358.

9. Courtney J. Riedinger et al., "Water Only Fasting and Its Effect on Chemotherapy Administration in Gynecologic Malignancies," *Gynecologic Oncology* 159, no. 3 (December 2020): 799–803, DOI:10.1016/j.ygyno.2020.09.008.

10. Stefanie de Groot et al., "Fasting-Mimicking Diet as an Adjunct to Neoadjuvant Chemotherapy for Breast Cancer in the Multicentre Randomized Phase 2 DIRECT Trial," *Nature Communications* 11, no. 1 (June 23, 2020): 3083, DOI:10.1038/s41467-020-16138-3.

11. Irene Caffa et al., "Author Correction: Fasting-Mimicking Diet and Hormone Therapy Induce Breast Cancer Regression," *Nature* 588, no. 7839 (December 2020): E33, DOI:10.1038/s41586-020-2957-6, erratum for Nature 583, no. 7817 (July 2020): 620–24.

12. Stefanie Zorn et al., "Impact of Modified Short-Term Fasting and Its Combination with a Fasting Supportive Diet During Chemotherapy on the Incidence and Severity of Chemotherapy-Induced Toxicities in Cancer Patients—a Controlled Cross-Over Pilot Study," *BMC Cancer* 20, no. 1 (June 22, 2020): 578, DOI:10.1186/s12885-020-07041-7.

13. Martin Voss et al., "ERGO2: A Prospective, Randomized Trial of Calorie-Restricted Ketogenic Diet and Fasting in Addition to Reirradiation for Malignant Glioma," *International Journal of Radiation Oncology, Biology, Physics* 108, no. 4 (November 15, 2020): 987–95, DOI:10.1016/j.ijrobp.2020.06.021.

14. Francesca Valdemarin et al., "Safety and Feasibility of Fasting-Mimicking Diet and Effects on Nutritional Status and Circulating Metabolic and Inflammatory Factors in Cancer Patients Undergoing Active Treatment," *Cancers* 13, no. 16 (August 9, 2021): 4013, DOI:10.3390/cancers13164013.

15. Karisa C. Schreck et al., "Feasibility and Biological Activity of a Ketogenic/Intermittent-Fasting Diet in Patients with Glioma," *Neurology* 97, no. 9 (August 31, 2021): e953–e963, DOI:10.1212/WNL.0000000000012386.

16. Claudio Vernieri et al., "Fasting-Mimicking Diet Is Safe and Reshapes Metabolism and Antitumor Immunity in Patients with Cancer," *Cancer Discovery* 12, no. 1 (January 2022): 90–107, DOI:10.1158/2159-8290.CD-21-0030.

17. Francesca Ligorio et al., "Exceptional Tumour Responses to Fasting-Mimicking Diet Combined with Standard Anticancer Therapies: A Sub-Analysis of the NCT03340935 Trial," *European Journal of Cancer* 172 (September 2022): 300–310, DOI:10.1016/j.ejca.2022.05.046.

18. Martin Voss et al., "Short-Term Fasting in Glioma Patients: Analysis of Diet Diaries and Metabolic Parameters of the ERGO2 Trial," *European Journal of Nutrition* 61, no. 1 (February 2022): 477–87, DOI:10.1007/s00394-021-02666-1.

INDEX